PHYSICS AND INSTRUMENTATION

Diagnostic Medical Ultrasound

Au

Ti

Du

SG

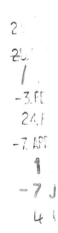

PHYSICS AND INSTRUMENTATION OF
Diagnostic Medical Ultrasound

PETER FISH

University of Wales–Bangor
School of Electronic Engineering Science

and

Gwynedd and Clwyd Health Authorities
Department of Medical Physics

JOHN WILEY & SONS
Chichester · New York · Brisbane · Toronto · Singapore

Reprinted June 1992, November 1994

Other Wiley Editorial Offices

John Wiley & Sons, Inc., 605 Third Avenue,
New York, NY 10158–0012, USA

Jacaranda Wiley Ltd, G.P.O. Box 859, Brisbane,
Queensland 4001, Australia

John Wiley & Sons (Canada) Ltd, 22 Worcester Road,
Rexdale, Ontario M9W 1L1, Canada

John Wiley & Sons (SEA) Pte Ltd, 37 Jalan Pemimpin 05–04,
Block B, Union Industrial Building, Singapore 2057

Library of Congress Cataloging-in-Publication Data:

Fish, Peter.
    Physics and instrumentation of diagnostic medical ultrasound /
Peter Fish.
        p.   cm.
    Includes bibliographical references.
    ISBN 0 471 92651 5
    1. Diagnosis, Ultrasonic. 2. Diagnosis, Ultrasonic—Instruments.
I. Title.
    [DNLM: 1. Ultrasonic Diagnosis—instrumentation. 2. Ultrasonic
Diagnosis—methods. 3. Ultrasonics.   WB 289 F532p]
RC78.7.U4F48 1990
616.07'543—dc20
DNLM/DLC
for Library of Congress   89-70688
                                                                CIP

British Library Cataloguing in Publication Data

Fish, Peter
    Physics and instrumentation of diagnostic medical ultrasound.
    1. Medicine. Diagnosis. Ultrasonography
    I. Title
    616.07'543

ISBN 0 471 92651 5

Phototypeset by Photo-graphics, Honiton, Devon.
Printed and bound in Great Britain by Redwood Books, Trowbridge, Wiltshire

To my family

Contents

CONTENTS

Preface

In any rapidly changing field there is a continual need for new texts. This is the author's excuse for yet another book on the physics of medical diagnostic ultrasound. There is inevitably an overlap with previous books, but there is much new material, and an emphasis reflecting the current state of the subject.

The goal has been to provide a text on the subject which is suitable for students requiring knowledge of the physics and instrumentation to complement and aid study of the clinical use of diagnostic ultrasound, whilst also being a useful introduction to the subject for those planning to investigate in greater depth.

It has also been a goal to provide a compact, reasonably priced text for personal use, rather than a library book. As a result, the presentation is deliberately condensed with an emphasis on descriptive line diagrams, in order to cover a wide subject in a short volume, without necessarily sacrificing depth.

I should like to thank Mrs Geraldine Park for typing the manuscript, Mr Tony Griffiths for drawing the illustrations, my family for their tolerance during the gestation period and my sonographer students, whose signs of a light dawning encouraged me to tackle this project.

CHAPTER 1

Introduction

1.1 ULTRASOUND

A sound or ultrasound wave consists of a mechanical disturbance of a medium (gas, liquid or solid) which passes through the medium at a fixed speed. Sound waves consist of a disturbance of air molecules, the vibrations of which pass from molecule to molecule from the speaker to the ear of the listener. Note that the molecules themselves do not move from speaker to listener—merely the disturbance. The rate at which particles in the medium vibrate in the disturbance is the frequency or pitch of the sound and is measured in hertz (cycles/second). As the pitch increases there comes a frequency at about 20 kHz when the sound is no longer audible and above this frequency the disturbance is known as ultrasound.

1.2 MEDICAL ULTRASOUND

In medical ultrasound, the disturbance, which is characterised by the local pressure change or distance of movement of the particles of the medium from their resting positions, originates at an electromechanical transducer in a probe placed on the skin surface. The transducer (operating as a transmitter) changes electrical signals to mechanical movement. The mechanical vibrations can be changed to electrical signals by the same transducer working in reverse (as a receiver). The ultrasound frequencies used are high—in the 1–20 MHz region—and are used to enable short pulses and narrow beams to be employed for accurate echo location.

The disturbance propagates through a medium at a speed which depends on the medium's compressibility and density. The speeds in different soft tissues vary slightly but are approximately 1540 m/s which leads to a transit time of 6.5 μs/cm.

1.3 PULSE–ECHO IMAGING

At a boundary between two tissues some ultrasound passes on and some is reflected in a similar fashion to that of light at a pane of glass. The degree of reflection depends on the acoustic impedances of the two tissues—again dependent on density and compressibility. A large difference in acoustic impedance leads to a high degree of reflection—for example at soft-tissue–bone or soft-tissue–air interfaces. At the boundary between two different types of soft tissue (e.g. muscle–fat) the degree of reflection is small. If the ultrasound is incident on a rough surface or on small objects then the ultrasound is scattered rather than reflected.

In ultrasonic imaging the transducer is periodically driven by an electrical pulse leading to the transmission of a pulse of ultrasound which is received back at the transducer after reflection or scatter at tissue interfaces. The time of arrival of the echo from a given interface depends on the depth of that interface and the instrument can use the time of arrival of an echo after transmission as an indication of the depth of the interface.

The transducer transmits and receives ultrasound along a pencil-like beam, the thickness of which is determined by the transducer's size, frequency of operation and any focussing arrangements. Thus if the instrument receives an echo it is known that the interface giving rise to the echo is within the ultrasound beam and the depth is given by the time of arrival of the echo after transmission. Clearly the orientation of the ultrasound beam and the time of arrival allow the location of the interface to be calculated and displayed.

Since the amplitude of an echo is determined by the structure and physical composition of the reflector or scatter, it is of diagnostic significance and is used to determine the brightness of display of the echo.

1.4 CHOICE OF FREQUENCY

Ultrasound is attenuated (loses energy) during its passage through tissue by scatter of the ultrasound outside the ultrasound beam, by partial reflection and by conversion into heat (absorption). Different tissues attenuate ultrasound to different degrees (e.g. muscle attenuates more strongly than fat). In addition, attenuation increases with frequency and the choice of ultrasound frequency is a compromise between the requirements of resolution (the ability to resolve close objects), which requires a high frequency, and penetration, which requires a low frequency. This compromise leads to the use of high frequencies for imaging superficial organs and lower frequencies for deeper structures.

1.5 A-SCAN

The simplest pulse–echo instrument is the A-scan device (Figure 1.1), which displays received echo amplitude as a graph against time. The depth of each reflector is indicated by the time of arrival of its echo.

1.6 B-SCAN

Two-dimensional images are generated by the B-scan instrument, in which the ultrasound beam is scanned through the tissue as shown in Figure 1.2. In earlier instruments the movement was accomplished by moving a single transducer by hand. Usually this movement is now achieved by motorised movement of a transducer, or by electronic beam steering, using a multi-element transducer.

The echo signals received at each beam position are displayed as spots on the display screen, the brightness indicating the echo amplitude (greyscale display). The position of the spots are determined by the orientation of the beam and by the time of arrival of the echoes.

1.7 REAL-TIME

Real-time scanners sweep the beam periodically through the region of interest at a sufficiently high rate—updating the image during each sweep—that tissue movement (e.g. heart valve or fetal movement) can be seen as it occurs.

1.8 M-MODE

The movement of echo-generating tissues can be displayed as a function of time by means of the M-mode (TM-mode) display. The change in reflector depth with time is displayed as shown in Figure 1.3. This allows the dynamics of heart valves to be measured.

1.9 DOPPLER

Movement of reflectors or scatterers also changes the frequency of the received signal. This change from the transmitted signal frequency is known as the Doppler effect and the magnitude of the change (Doppler shift) is proportional to the reflector or scatterer velocity. By measuring the Doppler shift in the ultrasound scattered from

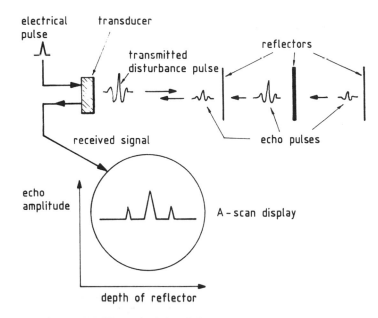

Figure 1.1 The principle of the ultrasonic A-scanner.

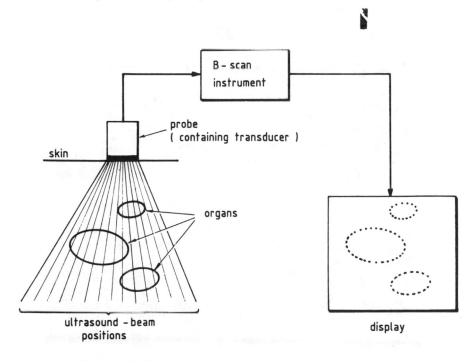

Figure 1.2 The principle of the ultrasonic B-scanner.

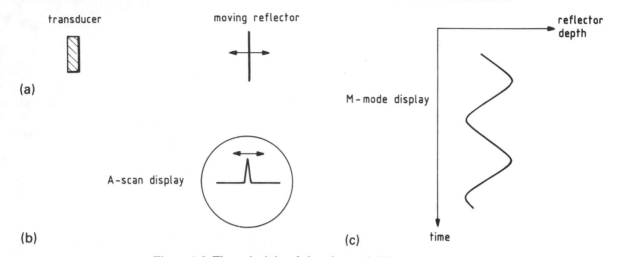

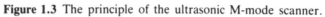

Figure 1.3 The principle of the ultrasonic M-mode scanner.

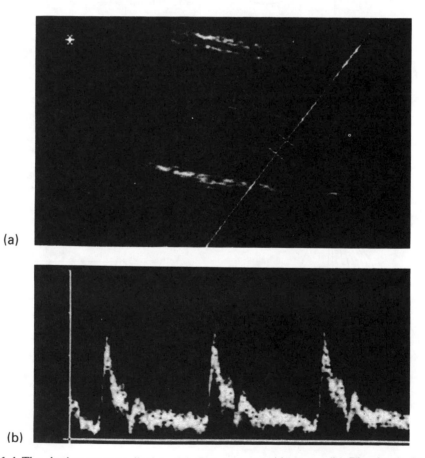

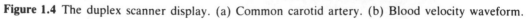

Figure 1.4 The duplex scanner display. (a) Common carotid artery. (b) Blood velocity waveform.

blood, the cyclical variation of blood velocity in arteries may be monitored and the disease-induced changes in velocity waveform or the increased range of Doppler shift frequencies from disturbed flow can be detected.

1.10 DUPLEX

Duplex scanners combining real-time scanners with Doppler effect instruments are used to display both vessel anatomy and blood velocity waveform simultaneously, as shown in Figure 1.4.

1.11 COLOURFLOW IMAGING

Colourflow imagers integrate the real-time and Doppler instruments still further and superimpose the image of moving blood, in colour, on the real-time greyscale display. Regions of disturbed flow may be indicated, together with direction and speed of blood flow, by appropriate colour coding.

CHAPTER 2

Nature of Ultrasound

2.1 INTRODUCTION

There are two types of wave motion—transverse and longitudinal. In transverse waves the disturbance is perpendicular to the direction of propagation. An example is surface waves on water. Longitudinal waves have the property that the disturbance is in the same direction as that of the propagation of the wave. Examples of longitudinal waves are sound and ultrasound waves. They are also called compressional waves. During the propagation of a disturbance, as the particles move in the same direction as the direction of propagation they move closer to their neighbours and compress the medium, causing a local increase in pressure. When, as a result of the elasticity of the medium, they move back in the opposite direction they move away from their neighbours and create a local rarefaction or reduction in local pressure. This change in pressure resulting from the passage of a disturbance is called the excess pressure.

2.2 CONTINUOUS WAVES

2.2.1 Period, Frequency and Wavelength

The surface of the source of continuous wave ultrasound will move in position in a sinusoidal fashion as shown in Figure 2.1. The period of the source (T) is the time between similar points on consecutive cycles of the waveform describing the source–surface position versus time and the frequency (f) of the source is the number of

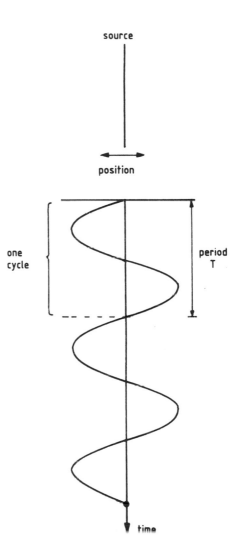

Figure 2.1 The continuous wave source–surface position variation with time.

cycles per second. The period and frequency are related by:

$$f = 1/T \qquad (2.1)$$

The motion of the source causes a similar motion of the particles of the medium thus at any position in front of the source the particles exhibit sinusoidally varying displacements away from their resting positions. The particle displacement, particle velocity and excess pressure at any point

in the medium in front of the source vary with time in a sinusoidal fashion, with the same frequency as the source, and are related to one another as shown in Figure 2.2. The maximum value of any of these quantities is known as its amplitude. Thus the excess pressure amplitude is P_0.

If we look at the variation of these quantities with distance from the source, at an instant in time (a snapshot), they appear as shown in Figure 2.3. The distance between similar points on

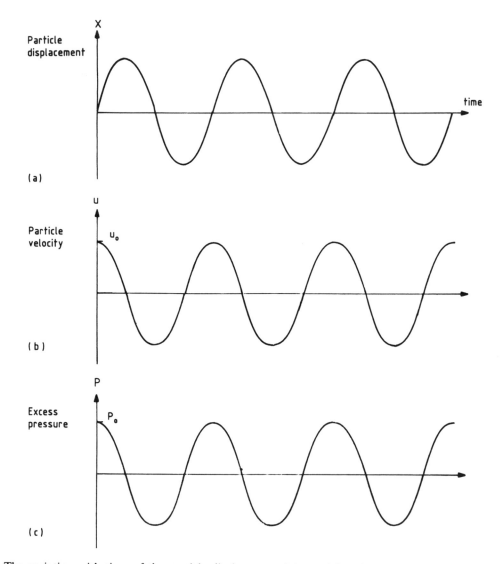

Figure 2.2 The variation with time of the particle displacement (a), particle velocity (b) and excess pressure (c) at a point in the medium in front of a source of continuous wave ultrasound.

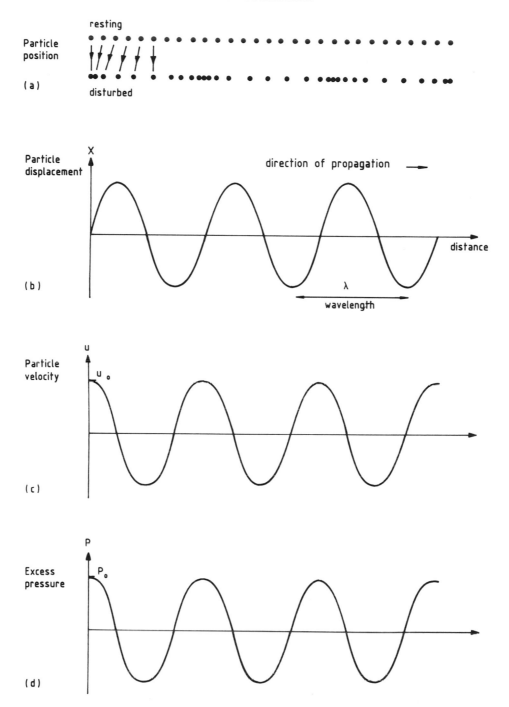

Figure 2.3 The positions of particles of a medium at rest and when disturbed by the passage of an ultrasonic wave (a), the particle displacement (b), particle velocity (c) and excess pressure (d), all shown as a variation with distance from the source at an instant in time. This is sometimes termed a 'snapshot' view.

consecutive cycles of the waveforms, in this case, is called the wavelength (λ). The disturbance must move distance λ in time T. Thus the wavelength and frequency are related to the speed of sound (c) by:

$$c = \lambda/T$$

$$= \lambda f \qquad (2.2)$$

2.2.2 Speed of Ultrasound

The disturbance moves at a fixed velocity in any one medium, the movement of one particle in the medium being passed to its neighbour through the forces of attraction between neighbouring particles. The speed of transmission of the ultrasound is dependent on the mass and spacing of the particles and the strength of the forces of attraction between the particles. This is illustrated in Figure 2.4. The speed of transmission increases as the strength of attraction between particles increases (i.e. c is higher for stiffer materials) and decreases as the mass of the particles increases

(the material becomes more dense). The exact relationship is shown below:

Speed of ultrasound

$$c = \sqrt{\frac{K}{\rho}} \qquad \text{m/s} \qquad (2.3)$$

or

$$c = \frac{1}{\sqrt{\kappa\rho}} \qquad \text{m/s} \qquad (2.4)$$

where
$$\rho = \text{density (kg/m}^3) \qquad (2.5)$$

$$K = \text{elastic modulus (stiffness)} = \frac{\text{stress}}{\text{strain}} \qquad (2.6)$$

$$= \frac{\text{excess pressure}}{\substack{\text{fractional change} \\ \text{in volume}}} \quad (\text{kg m}^{-1}\,\text{s}^{-2})$$

and $\quad \kappa = 1/K = \text{compressibility}$

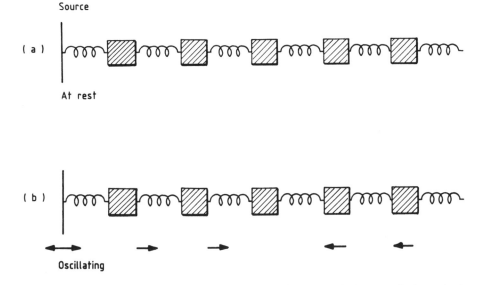

Figure 2.4 A simple model of the particles of a medium in front of a source of ultrasound where the intermolecular forces of attraction are shown as springs. The configurations at rest (a) and with an oscillating source (b) are shown.

Examples of velocities in various biological media are shown in Table 2.1.

Table 2.1.

Medium	Velocity (m/s)
Air	330
Water (20°C)	1480
Blood	1570
Fat	1460
Muscle	1580
Bone	3500
Soft tissue (mean)	1540

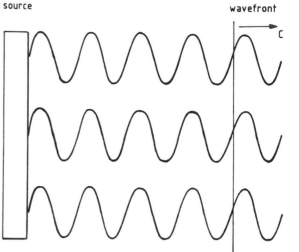

Figure 2.5 A plane wavefront.

2.2.3 Tissue Impedance

The velocity of the particles of the medium is related to the excess pressure by a quantity called the tissue impedance. The impedance is determined again by tissue density and compressibility and can be calculated from the density and propagation velocity as shown below:

$$Z = \frac{\text{Excess pressure}}{\text{Particle velocity}} = \frac{P_0}{U_0} \quad (2.7)$$

It is usually calculated from

$$Z = \rho c = \sqrt{\frac{\rho}{\kappa}} \quad \text{rayls or kg m}^{-2} \text{ s}^{-1} \quad (2.8)$$

2.2.4 Wavefronts

A source of ultrasound emits from all points on its active surface and ultrasound is present throughout a volume in front of the source. The surface joining similar points on a similar cycle (as shown in Figure 2.5) is known as a wavefront. The direction of travel of the ultrasound is perpendicular to the wavefront, which moves forward at the ultrasound velocity. Figure 2.5 shows an example of a plane wavefront. Figure 2.6 shows the wavefronts emitted from plane and focussed transducers. Close to a plane transducer, the wavefronts are approximately plane, but further away, the beam starts to diverge and the wavefronts become increasingly convex until, far from the source, each wavefront forms part of a spherical surface. The wavefronts from a focussed transducer are concave close to the transducer when the beam is converging, plane in the focal region and convex in the diverging portion of the beam distal to the focal region.

2.2.5 Energy, Power and Intensity

Electrical energy (measured in joules) is used to drive the transducer and is converted into mechanical energy. This mechanical energy, when absorbed in the tissue, can generate heat. The rate of generation, or passage of energy, is called the power of the source or beam and is measured in joules/sec or watts. The power is confined to different cross-sectional areas, depending on the width of the ultrasound beam. For example, objects of similar size placed at points A and B in the beam illustrated in Figure 2.7 receive different powers, even though they are the same

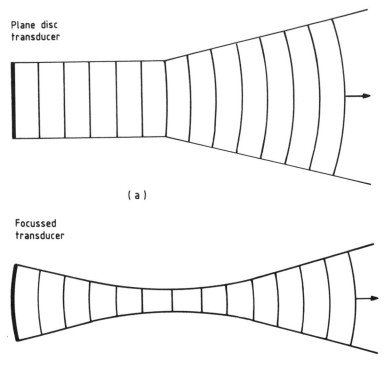

Figure 2.6 The wavefronts, at an instant, from a plane disc transducer (a) and a focussed transducer (b).

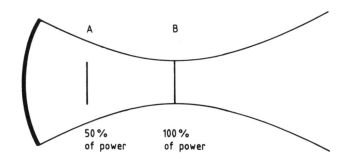

Figure 2.7 The percentage of transmitted power crossing two similar areas at different positions in a focussed beam.

size and even though the total powers passing through the beam at points A and B are the same. This is solely because the ultrasound power is more concentrated at B than it is at A. The concept of intensity allows us to take this effect into account. The ultrasound intensity is the power passing through unit area, perpendicular to the direction of propagation. The intensity is proportional to the product of excess pressure and particle velocity and is given by the expressions below:

$$\text{Intensity } I = \frac{1}{2} P_0 U_0 \quad \text{W/m}^2$$

$$= \frac{1}{2} P_0^2/Z \quad \text{W/m}^2 \qquad (2.9)$$

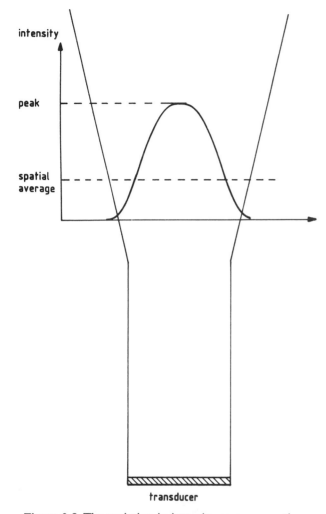

Figure 2.8 The variation in intensity across a continuous wave ultrasound beam showing the peak and spatial average intensities.

The intensity is not uniform across the ultrasound beam but generally peaks towards the centre of the beam and reduces towards the outside as illustrated in Figure 2.8. An average intensity of the ultrasound beam can be calculated by averaging the intensity over the cross-sectional area of the beam—the limits of which are often taken to be a fixed small fraction (e.g. 10%) of the peak intensity. This average over the beam cross-section is known as the spatial average.

2.3 PULSED WAVES

2.3.1 Pulse Shapes

Continuous wave ultrasound is used in some Doppler instruments and therapy instruments but in the main, medical ultrasound makes use of pulses. Typical variations of ultrasound excess pressure with time for imaging, pulse Doppler and therapy applications are shown in Figure 2.9. Imaging applications require short pulses in order to easily separate the echoes from nearby reflectors. A typical imaging pressure pulse will be 1–3 cycles long. A pulsed Doppler waveform used to obtain signals from flowing blood will typically be 1–20 μs long. Therapy machines are often pulsed, but in this case the pulses are extremely long (approximately 2 ms) and the off time between pulses will frequently be not dissimilar (2–8 ms). The reason for pulsing therapy machines is to reduce thermal effects by allowing some cooling between pulses.

The time variation of pressure shown in Figure 2.10b results from the pressure pulse shown in Figure 2.10a passing through a fixed point (distance D_1) at a constant velocity. Note that the waveform shown as a function of time is a reversal of the waveform shown as a function of distance.

2.3.2 Intensity

With pulsed ultrasound, the intensity not only has a spatial variation but also varies with time. The variation of excess pressure and intensity at a point in the beam is shown in Figure 2.11. The intensity is proportional to the square of the excess pressure (equation 2.9). The maximum intensity in this case is called the temporal peak and the average taken over time, the temporal average. The combined effect of a variation in excess pressure with distance and time is illustrated in Figure 2.12. The pressure pulse from the transducer moves along the ultrasound beam at a fixed rate. At any instant the variations in intensity along the beam and across the beam are as shown in Figure 2.12a. If the spatial peak

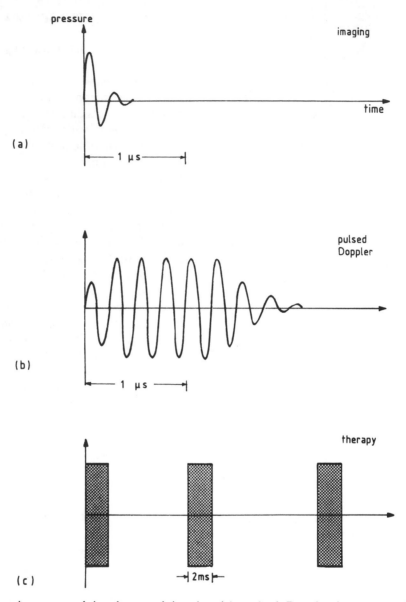

Figure 2.9 Typical pulses as used in ultrasound imaging (a), pulsed Doppler instruments (b) and therapy instruments (c).

intensity is monitored at the highest intensity part of the beam then the variation will be as shown in Figure 2.12b and the peak of this waveform will be the spatial peak, temporal peak intensity (I_{sptp}). If this waveform is averaged over time, then it is termed the spatial peak temporal average intensity (I_{spta}). If the spatial average intensity is monitored (Figure 2.12c) then the waveform will have a similar shape but lower amplitude and the average value of this waveform will be the spatial average temporal average (I_{sata}). The importance of these quantities will be discussed in the chapter on bioeffects, dosimetry and safety.

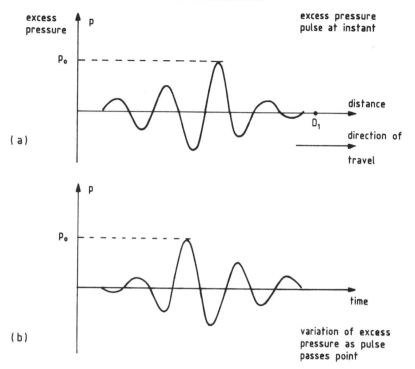

Figure 2.10 The pulsed ultrasound excess pressure variation with distance at an instant in time (a) and the variation with time at a particular point in the ultrasound field (b).

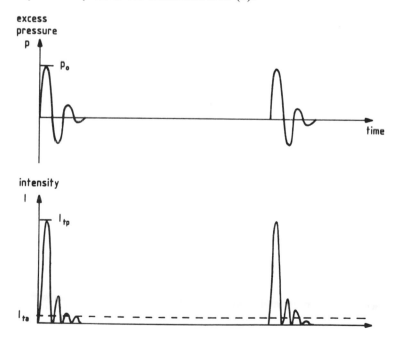

Figure 2.11 The excess pressure and intensity variation with time at a point in the field of a repetitively pulsed ultrasound source showing the temporal peak (I_{tp}) and temporal average (I_{ta}) intensities.

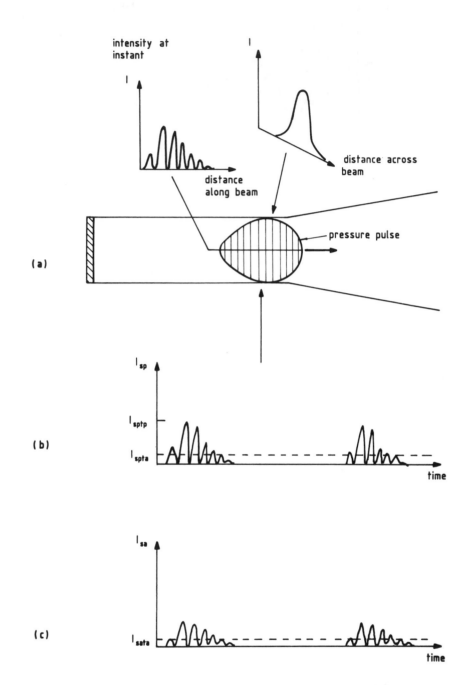

Figure 2.12 (a) The wavefronts of a pressure pulse in the field of a plane ultrasound transducer at an instant in time, together with the intensity variation along the beam axis and across the beam. (b) The time variation of the spatial peak intensity (I_{sp})—the intensity at the position in the beam at which the intensity is a maximum, showing the spatial peak, temporal peak (I_{sptp}) and spatial peak temporal average (I_{spta}) values. (c) The time variation of the spatial average (I_{sa}) and its temporal average value (I_{sata}).

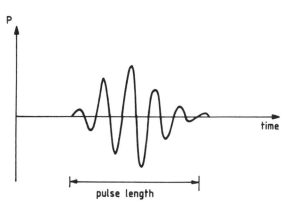

Figure 2.13 The length (duration) of an ultrasound pulse.

2.3.3 Pulse Length

The duration of an ultrasound pressure pulse is commonly called the pulse length, as illustrated in Figure 2.13. The limits of the pulse need to be fairly carefully defined in order to give a figure to the pulse length. For example, it might be the length of the pulse contained within limits of half-cycles, exceeding the threshold of 10% of the maximum half-cycle amplitude.

2.3.4 Energy

Each of the emitted pulses contains a certain energy and therefore the energy emitted per second or the average transmitted power is equal to the pulse energy multiplied by the pulse repetition frequency (PRF). The total energy emitted by the transducer in time T_{On} is the average transmitted power multiplied by T_{On}.

2.3.5 Frequency Spectrum

Waveforms can be synthesised by adding together sinusoidal waves of differing frequencies. This is illustrated in Figure 2.14 where the waveform at the bottom of the figure has been synthesised by adding together the five sinusoidal waveforms at the top. Altering the number of waveforms, their range of frequencies, the amplitude of the various components, and their time relationship will alter the resultant waveform shape. Any waveform can be synthesised in this way. Conversely, it is possible to consider any particular waveform as equivalent to a range of sinusoidal waves of differing frequencies. The frequency components comprising the waveform in Figure 2.14 are shown on the right-hand side of Figure 2.15a. The horizontal axis gives the frequency of the component and the height of the line representing that component indicates its amplitude. The frequency components comprising waveforms found in practice can be considered to be so close together as to form a continuous variation with frequency and examples of the 'frequency spectrum' for two different pulse waveforms are shown in Figure 2.15b and c. The width of the frequency spectrum is known as the bandwidth of the pulse. It can be seen from the illustration that the bandwidth increases as the pulse length decreases. In fact they are inversely proportional. The nominal frequency of the pulse is usually measured as the 'zero crossing frequency', which is the frequency of the sine wave which has the same number of crossings on the time axis per unit time as the pulse. The zero crossing frequency will normally be approximately the mid-point frequency of the spectrum. Thus pulses can be said to have a frequency (zero crossing frequency) and bandwidth (the width of their frequency spectrum—usually taken as the width at half the maximum).

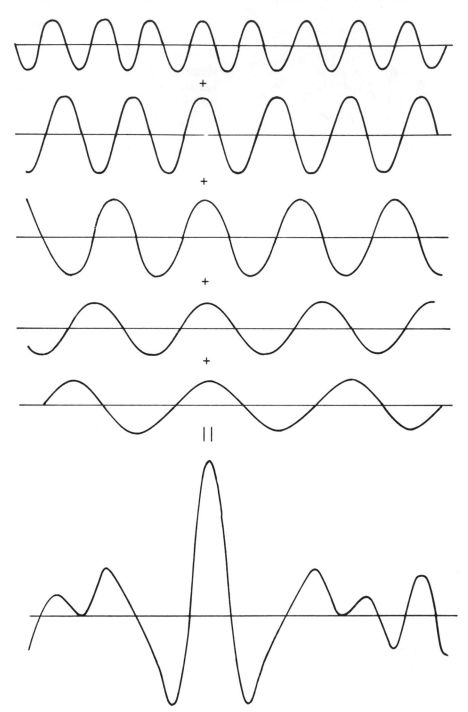

Figure 2.14 Synthesis of a pulse waveform from the addition of sine waves of different frequencies, amplitudes and phases (see Section 4.1.1). Conversely, a pulse waveform may be analysed (broken down) in terms of sine waves covering a range of frequencies.

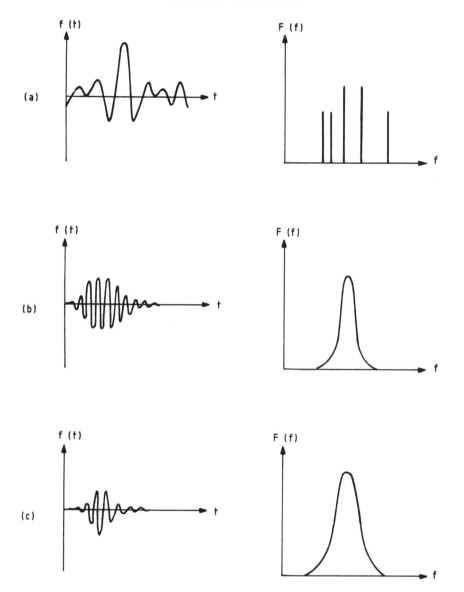

Figure 2.15 The frequency spectra corresponding to various pulse waveforms. (a) The case considered in Figure 2.14, (b) a long pulse and (c) a short pulse. The width of the spectrum (the range of frequencies needed to synthesise the pulse) is inversely proportional to the duration of the pulse.

CHAPTER 3

Propagation in Tissue

3.1 INTRODUCTION

Ultrasound is altered by the tissue through which it passes. At the boundaries between different tissue types, it is partially reflected and can be bent by refraction, it is scattered from the main beam by small tissue structures and it loses energy by absorption. These effects are important in the consideration of instrument design, and understanding and avoiding artifacts.

3.2 SPECULAR REFLECTION

When ultrasound is incident on a smooth boundary (interface) between two media some ultrasound is transmitted through the interface and some reflected. If the interface is perpendicular to the direction of propagation (Figure 3.1) then the intensities of the ultrasound beams reflected

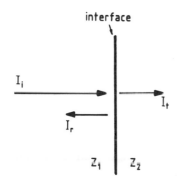

Figure 3.1 The incident (I_i), transmitted (I_t) and reflected (I_r) intensities at a plane interface between media of acoustic impedances Z_1 and Z_2.

(I_r) and transmitted (I_t) at the interface, expressed as a fraction of the incident beam intensity (I_i), are governed by the acoustic impedances of the two media as shown below:

$$R = \frac{I_r}{I_i} = \frac{(Z_2 - Z_1)^2}{(Z_1 + Z_2)^2} \qquad (3.1)$$

$$T = \frac{I_t}{I_i} = \frac{4Z_1Z_2}{(Z_1 + Z_2)^2} \qquad (3.2)$$

where

R = Intensity reflection coefficient $\qquad$ (3.3)
$T = (1-R)$ = Intensity transmission coefficient

When the ultrasound is incident on the surface at a non-zero angle to the perpendicular at the surface, as shown in Fig. 3.2, the reflected and transmitted intensities are dependent not only on the acoustic impedances but also on the angle of incidence. In all cases of specular reflection the angle of incidence (θ_i) equals the angle of reflection (θ_r).

$$\theta_i = \theta_r \qquad (3.4)$$

Note that these angles are measured to the perpendicular to the interface and not to the interface itself.

3.3 REFRACTION

The transmitted beam at an interface between media having different speeds of ultrasound

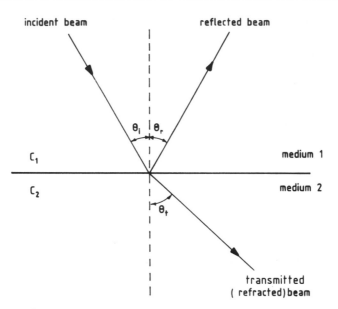

Figure 3.2 The incident, reflected and transmitted (refracted) beams at the interface between media with characteristic velocities (c_1 and c_2). The angle of incidence is θ_i, the angle of reflection is θ_r and the angle of refraction is θ_t.

deviates from the path of incident beam provided the angle of incidence is non-zero (Figure 3.2). The relationship between the angle of incidence and the angle of refraction (θ_t) and the velocities in the two media (c_1 and c_2) is given by Snell's Law:

$$\frac{\sin \theta_t}{\sin \theta_i} = \frac{c_2}{c_1} \qquad (3.5)$$

Note that the beam deviation is dependent on the difference of the ultrasound speeds (not impedances) and the refracted beam bends away from the perpendicular if the speed in the second medium is higher than in the first and *vice versa*.

3.4 NON-SPECULAR REFLECTION AND SCATTER

If ultrasound is incident on a rough surface or on particles with a size small or comparable with a wavelength then the ultrasound is scattered

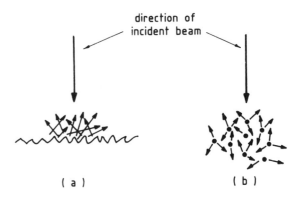

Figure 3.3 Scatter from (a) a rough surface and (b) a distribution of small targets.

in all directions (Figure 3.3). Generally the ultrasound power lost from the beam (scattered power) increases with frequency and, in particular, if the scattering particles are small compared with the wavelength then the scattered power is proportional to the fourth power of the ultrasound frequency.

3.5 ABSORPTION

Ultrasound is also lost from the beam by absorption in which the energy of the ultrasound is converted into heat. Again the loss due to absorption increases with frequency.

Absorption results from relaxation mechanisms which may be described as follows. All substances contain a certain amount of potential energy. This can be mechanical energy when the substance is under compression or tension; chemical energy, where the chemical bonding of molecules to form particular substances can alter with the absorption or release of energy; and structural energy concerned with the particular configuration of molecules, which again can be changed with the absorption or release of energy. All these energy states are linked and changes in one will affect the others. During compression of tissue during the passage of an ultrasound wave, some of the mechanical potential energy will convert into other energy states, thereby 'relaxing' the potential energy of compression. During the rarefaction half of the cycle the energy can convert back into mechanical energy. There are time delays involved in moving from one energy state to another. If the frequency is low, energy can move from the mechanical form into another during compression and back again during rarefaction and there is no net energy loss and therefore no absorption. At high frequencies, there is insufficient time for energy to change state during compression or rarefaction because these conditions do not last long enough, and there again there is no energy loss and no absorption. There is a range of frequencies over which some energy can move into another state, during compression, but not have time to completely move back again during rarefaction and over this range of frequencies there will be a net energy transfer and therefore absorption.

Conversion of energy from mechanical to heat by fluid friction or 'viscous energy loss' was thought to be a separate absorption mechanism. It is now considered to be within the relaxation mechanism category.

The variation of absorption coefficient with

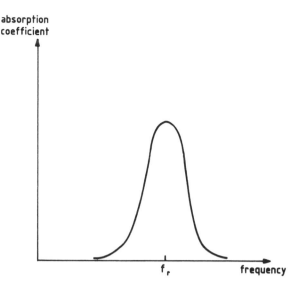

Figure 3.4 Variation of absorption coefficient with frequency for a single relaxation mechanism. The relaxation frequency is f_r.

frequency for one relaxation mechanism is shown in Figure 3.4. The frequency at which the absorption is a maximum is called the relaxation frequency for this particular mechanism. Biological tissues are particularly complex structures, and a large number of overlapping relaxation mechanisms, all with different relaxation frequencies, are involved. In general, the higher the relaxation frequency, the greater the absorption, and the variation in net absorption coefficient when there are a number of relaxation mechanisms involved increases with frequency as shown in Figure 3.5.

3.6 ATTENUATION

Attenuation is the reduction in ultrasound intensity during its passage through medium.

The attenuation mechanisms are shown below:

(1) Absorption (tissue specific).
(2) Scatter (tissue specific).
(3) Beam divergence.
(4) Reflection.
(5) Refraction?

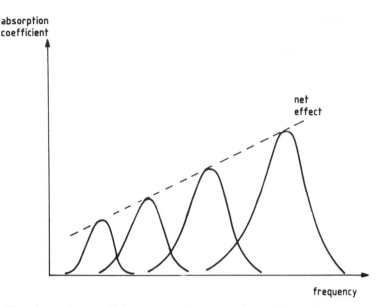

Figure 3.5 The absorption coefficient versus frequency for multiple relaxation mechanisms.

The reason for having some doubt as to whether refraction should be included as an attenuation mechanism is that if the whole beam is refracted at a tissue interface, then it cannot be said that the process involves any loss of intensity. On the other hand, refraction at the boundaries of structures of less than the beam diameter in lateral dimensions, and tissue inhomogeneities, will remove ultrasound from the beam and therefore lead to a loss of intensity.

Both specular and non-specular reflection reduce the intensity of ultrasound in its passage across a tissue interface.

Although the total power is unchanged as a beam diverges, it is contained within an increasing beam cross-sectional area and therefore the intensity decreases. This is sometimes called geometric attenuation. Beam convergence between a transducer and its focus causes an increase in intensity and could be considered negative geometric attenuation.

If we use a beam with plane wavefronts (non-diverging or converging beam) and a uniform sample of tissue (no boundaries at which reflection and refraction can take place) then attenuation is due solely to absorption and scatter and we can give a figure to the tissue to quantify its ability to attenuate ultrasound. The tissue attenuation coefficient (α) is the fractional rate of change of intensity with distance under these conditions:

$$\alpha = \frac{\Delta I}{I \Delta x} \quad \text{m}^{-1} \tag{3.6}$$

where ΔI is the loss of intensity from incident intensity I during passage through a thin layer of thickness Δx and where $\Delta I/I \ll 1$ (small change of intensity).

The change of intensity with distance for high and low attenuation coefficients is shown in Figure 3.6. Note that they are not straight lines because it is the fractional rate of change of intensity which is constant and not the absolute rate of change.

The equation describing the change of intensity with depth is:

$$I = I_0 e^{-\alpha x} \tag{3.7}$$

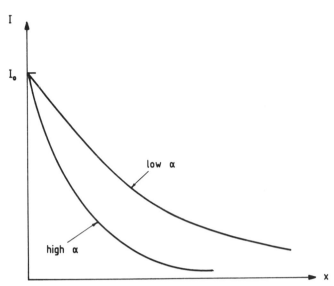

Figure 3.6 The variation in intensity with depth for media having low and high attenuation coefficients.

where

I = Intensity at depth x

I_0 = Intensity at depth zero

α = attenuation coefficient

= $\alpha_a + \alpha_s$ (absorption plus
scattering coefficients)   (3.8)

The units of α are m^{-1} or cm^{-1} when x is measured in metres or centimetres respectively.

The overall attenuation coefficient is the sum of the absorption and the scatter coefficients. Since the fractional change in intensity is a ratio it can be expressed in decibels (see Appendix B) and we can define a decibel attenuation coefficient given below:

$$\mu = 4.3\alpha \quad \text{dB/m} \quad (3.9)$$

The attenuation coefficient is very roughly proportional to frequency and is frequently given in the form shown below:

$$\mu \simeq kf \quad (3.10)$$

where k is in dB m^{-1} MHz^{-1} or the value of μ at 1 MHz and f is the frequency in MHz.

It should be noted that this is a very crude approximation and although there is an increase of attenuation with frequency for all tissues, the

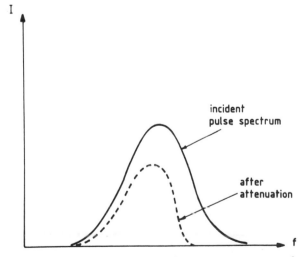

Figure 3.7 The change in the frequency spectrum of an ultrasound pulse as a result of frequency-dependent attenuation.

actual dependence on frequency can vary quite markedly from the relationship indicated above. Typical attenuation coefficients are shown in Table 3.1.

The dependence of attentuation on frequency has an effect on pulse spectrum shape and therefore on the shape of the ultrasound pulse itself. As shown in Figure 3.7, the high-frequency components of the ultrasound spectrum are attenuated far more strongly than the lower frequency components and therefore the mean frequency of the spectrum decreases and the spectral width decreases, leading to an increase in pulse length (see Section 2.3.5) and thereby to poorer axial resolution.

Table 3.1 Attenuation coefficient at 1 MHz dB m^{-1}.

Blood	20
Fat	60
Muscle	180
Liver	90
Soft tissue (mean)	70

CHAPTER 4

Beam Shapes and Transducers

4.1 PHASE AND INTERFERENCE

Before examining the shape of ultrasound beams, we need to understand the concepts of phase and interference.

4.1.1 Phase

The position or time in a cycle of a sinusoidally varying quantity is known as the phase and is measured in degrees. The reason for this can be seen from Figure 4.1. A sinusoid is the projection onto the y axis of a line of constant length R as a function of the angle (phase angle) between the line and the x axis. Different waves of the same frequency can be described as having a certain phase relationship measured in degrees. Figure 4.2 shows examples of waves which are 180 and 90 degrees out of phase with respect to the first shown waveform.

4.1.2 Interference

The importance of phase relationships can be seen as we consider the summation of waves. For example, the addition of waves which are in

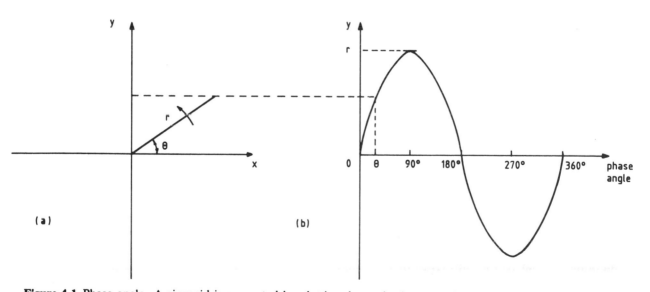

Figure 4.1 Phase angle. A sinusoid is generated by plotting the projection onto the y axis of a line of constant length (r) rotating about the origin against the angle of rotation (θ). The position of a point within a single cycle of a sinusoid can therefore be specified in terms of a phase angle between 0 and 360 degrees.

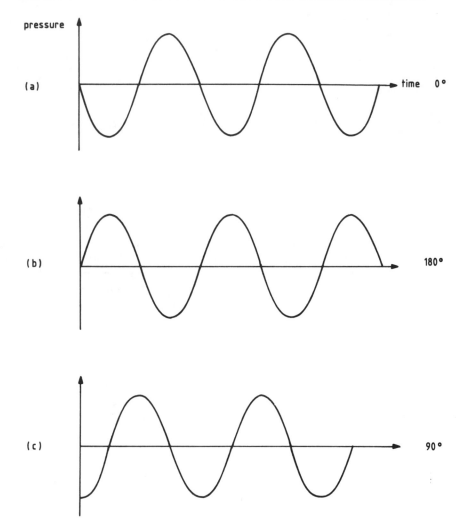

Figure 4.2 Phase difference. Sinusoidally varying quantities of the same frequency can have different phases at an instant. At any time the waveform in (b) is 180 degrees phase advanced on waveform (a). Waveform (c) is 90 degrees phase advanced on waveform (a).

phase leads to a wave which has an amplitude equal to the sum of the amplitudes of the two summed waves (constructive interference) whereas the resultant wave when two waves which are 180 degrees out of phase are added has an amplitude equal to the difference of the amplitudes of the summed waves (destructive interference). This is shown in Figure 4.3. Clearly there are intermediate resultant amplitudes for intermediate phase relationships.

4.2 BEAM SHAPE

The shape of ultrasound beams is determined by interference and Huygen's principle.

4.2.1 Huygen's Principle and Diffraction

Huygen's principle states that every point along a wavefront is itself a point source emitting a

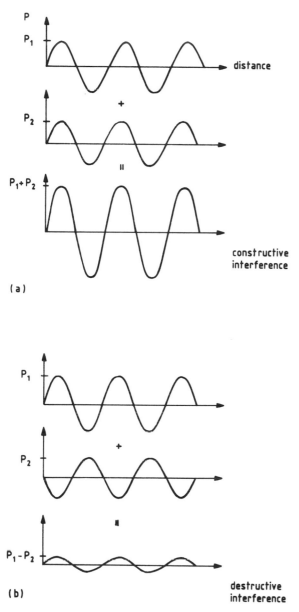

Figure 4.3 Constructive (a) and destructive (b) interference.

wave as shown in Figure 4.4 can be calculated by summing the contributions at each point in the field from all those points across the aperture. The wavelets from two points on the aperture are shown in the figure. There will be constructive interference at those points where the wavelet fronts are coincident. If this calculation is carried out, we find that the wavefronts on the far side of the aperture take the form shown in Figure 4.5. The wavefronts continue plane for a short distance from the aperture and then become more convex, leading to beam divergence, and closely approximate parts of spherical surfaces centred on the aperture when the wavefront is far from the aperture. The point at which the beam starts to diverge and the degree of divergence are dependent on the ratio of the aperture dimensions to the wavelength of the ultrasound. The important point to note is that there is bending of the ultrasound beam into the geometric shadow of the aperture and this phenomenon is called diffraction. It will also take place at a single edge and there will be bending in the opposite direction into the geometric shadow of a reflecting or absorbing object of less than the beam width. It should be noted that Figure 4.5 does not show variations in intensity, merely the extent of the beam containing most of the ultrasound power.

4.2.2 Transducer Beam Shape

The principle can be extended to the wavefronts from transducers and examples of the wavefronts from two disc transducers with different diameters are shown in Figure 4.6. In general, as the ratio of radius to wavelength increases, the distance from the transducer at which the beam begins to diverge increases and the degree of divergence decreases.

By considering the sum of the Huygen's wavelets emanating from all points on a transducer surface, we can calculate the variation of pressure and intensity in the ultrasound beam from a transducer. The case of the thin disc transducer of radius a is illustrated in Figure 4.7. Most of the ultrasound power is contained within

spherical wave. This means that the wave motion at any other point in an ultrasound field can be calculated by adding the contributions from spherical wavelets from all points on a particular wavefront. For example, the ultrasound field on the far side of an aperture insonated by a plane

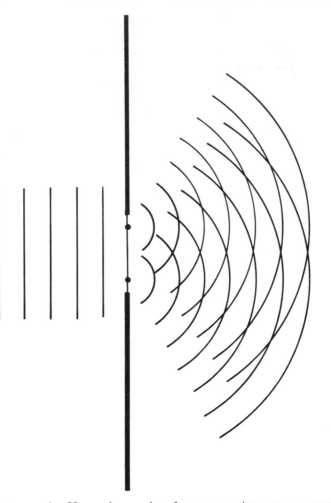

Figure 4.4 Interference between the Huygen's wavelets from two points on an aperture insonated by plane waves.

the surface (circular cylinder in the near zone and cone in the far zone) shown in longitudinal section in Figure 4.7a. The wavefronts are approximately plane and therefore the beam is non-diverging up to a distance determined by the transducer diameter and wavelength, and then diverges at an angle determined again by the ratio of the transducer diameter to wavelength. The half-angle of beam divergence θ is given by:

$$\sin \theta = 0.6\lambda/a \qquad (4.1)$$

If we plot the intensity along the axis of the ultrasound beam against distance then we find a wide variation of intensity within the non-diverging or near zone (Fresnel zone) and a gradual reduction in intensity within the diverging or far zone (Fraunhofer zone). The position of the last maximum of the axial intensity corresponds to the point at which the beam starts to diverge and its distance from the transducer is often known as the distance to the last axial maximum. This distance (Z_m) is given by:

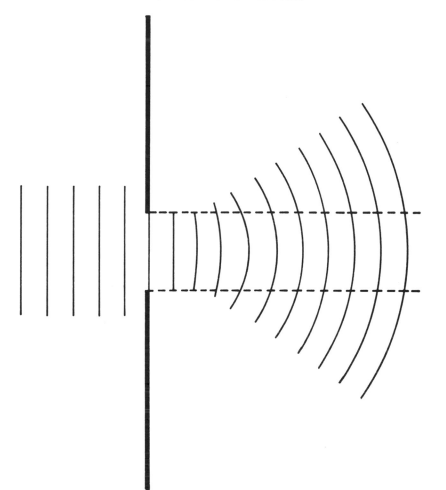

Figure 4.5 The wavefronts and beam shape from an aperture insonated by plane waves.

$$Z_m = a^2/\lambda \qquad (4.2)$$

The intensity only reaches zero within the Fresnel zone for a perfect disc transducer with a uniform velocity of movement over its surface. In practice, even with disc transducers, slight inhomogeneities within the transducer, variations in the backing material over the transducer surface and the attachment of wires to the electrodes on the transducer cause non-uniformities in surface velocity and in this case the variations along the

axis and elsewhere in the ultrasound beam are not so marked. The beam shape for rectangular transducers is qualitatively similar.

4.2.3 Side Lobes

Although the surface shown in Figure 4.7a contains most of the ultrasound intensity, there is often significant ultrasound energy outside this surface. The variation of intensity, particularly in

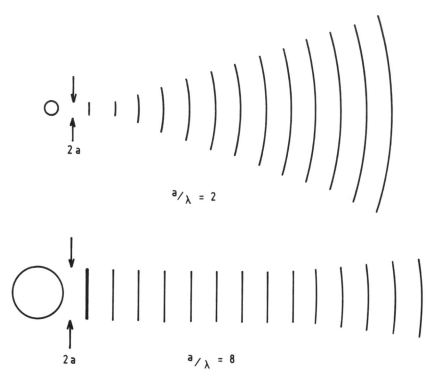

Figure 4.6 The wavefronts and beam shape from a plane disc transducer illustrating the dependence of beam shape on the ratio of radius to wavelength (a/λ).

the far field, is often illustrated by a polar intensity graph as shown in Figure 4.8. In this case the length of the line from the origin indicates the intensity (I) measured at the angle θ from the beam axis. It can be seen that most of the ultrasound power is contained within a main lobe, the extent of which would correspond to the surface shown in Figure 4.7a, but there are smaller side lobes present outside this surface. We shall see later when discussing artifacts that the side lobes can give rise to spurious images on the ultrasound screen and measures are often taken to reduce them.

4.2.4 Focussing

In order to achieve a narrower beam width than that achievable with a plane transducer, we make use of focussing. In order to achieve this we need to form the wavefronts into a concave shape so that they converge to a focus as shown in Figure 4.9. The wavefronts are converging between the transducer and the focal zone, approximately plane within the focal zone and then convex or diverging distal to the focus. As illustrated, one method of focussing is to form the transducer into part of the surface of a sphere. The degree of focussing depends on the radius of curvature of the transducer (Figure 4.10) and the position of the last axial maxima of the equivalent plane transducer. The ranges of the ratio of the distance to the last axial maximum to the radius of the curvature for weak, medium and strong focussing are shown in Figure 4.11.

It should be noted that it is only possible to get a useful narrowing of the ultrasound beam in the near zone and the beginning of the far zone,

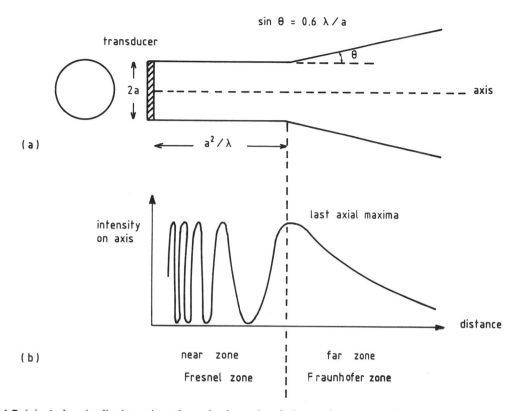

Figure 4.7 (a) A longitudinal section through the axis of the surface containing most of the power in an ultrasound beam from a circular transducer of radius a. (b) The variation in intensity along the beam axis.

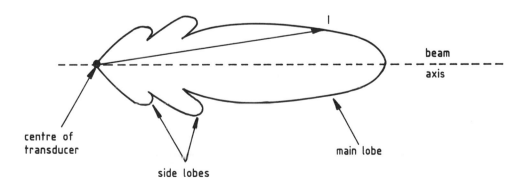

Figure 4.8 The beam intensity plotted in polar co-ordinates.

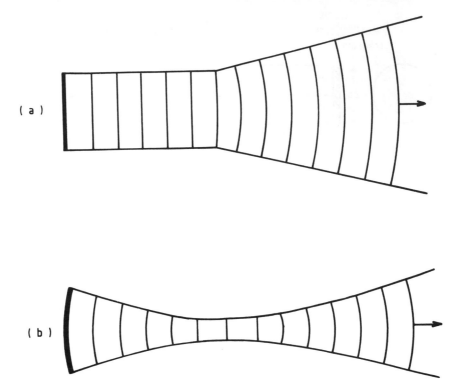

Figure 4.9 The wavefronts and beam shape of a plane disc transducer (a) and bowl-shaped focussed transducer (b).

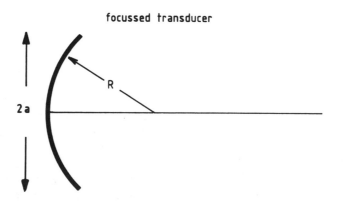

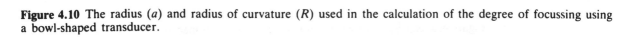

Figure 4.10 The radius (*a*) and radius of curvature (*R*) used in the calculation of the degree of focussing using a bowl-shaped transducer.

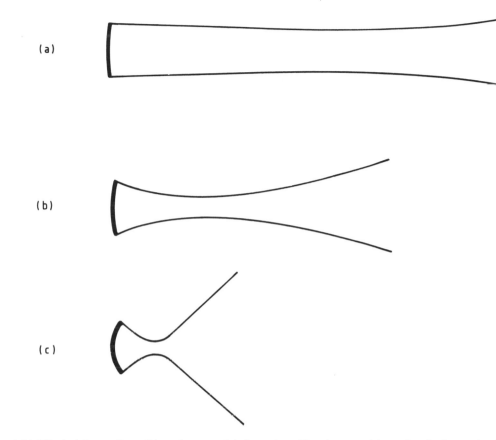

(a)

(b)

(c)

Figure 4.11 Weak (a), medium (b) and strong (c) focussing. The degree of focussing is determined by the ratio of the near zone length (Z_m) to the radius of curvature (R).

Weak focussing:	$2 \geqslant Z_m/R > 0$
Medium focussing:	$2\pi \geqslant Z_m/R > 2$
Strong focussing:	$Z_m/R > 2\pi$

since we are going to have diffraction spread of the ultrasound beam when we are well into the far zone, whatever the degree of focussing. Also, increasing the strength of focussing by reducing the radius of curvature of the transducer will give a narrower beam at the focus but the useful length of narrowed beam (length of focal zone) will decrease. The width and length of the focal zone are illustrated in Figure 4.12. There is a simple formula for the width and this is given in the figure.

Focussing not only decreases the width of the ultrasound beam but also increases the intensity of the beam at the focus as a result of concentrating the power of the beam within a smaller area. Plots of axial intensity against distance from a transducer are shown in Figure 4.13. It should be noted that the maximum intensity is not at the radius of curvature but is between that point and the transducer.

Forming the transducer into a bowl shape is only one way of achieving a focussing action. Alternative methods are the use of a lens and a mirror as shown in Figure 4.14. Note the use of a concave-surfaced lens for focussing using ultrasound as opposed to the convex surface

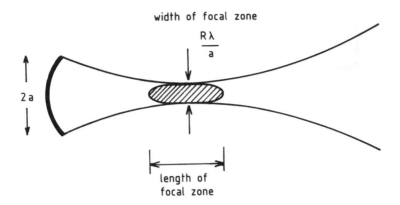

Figure 4.12 The focal zone.

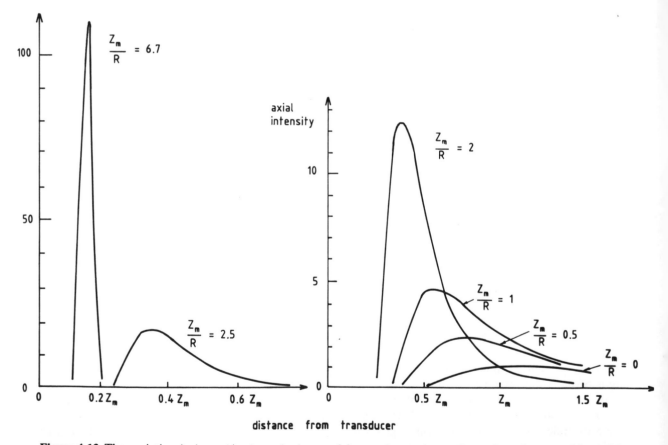

distance from transducer

Figure 4.13 The variation in intensity along the beam of focussed transducers for various degrees of focussing. Reprinted with permission from *Ultrasound in Medicine and Biology*, **5**, Kossof, G., Analysis of focussing action of spherically curved transducers, © 1979 Pergamon Press PLC.

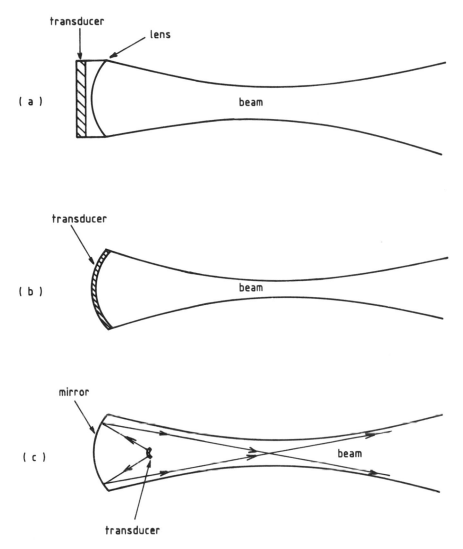

Figure 4.14 Focussing by (a) lens, (b) transducer shaping and (c) concave mirror.

used in optical lenses. The focussing action is dependent on the refraction of the ultrasound at the lens surface and convergence of the emerging beam results from a higher velocity of ultrasound in the lens than in tissue. The lens is usually made of a plastic or hard rubber material. The mirror transducer arrangement is used in a water or oil bath.

4.2.5 Pulsed Beam Shapes

We have considered beam shapes and focussing in the context of continuous wave ultrasound. The beam shape and focussing action will be slightly different when using pulsed ultrasound. In general, the variation in intensity, particularly in the near zone and the side lobes in the far zone, will be reduced as the pulse length becomes shorter. The reason for this is that the pulses have a bandwidth, that is to say they can be considered as the summation of continuous waves of a range of frequencies. The interference maxima and minima arising from each frequency component are in different positions in the ultrasound beam and when added up tend to smooth out the variations. In addition, the position, width and length of the focal zone are dependent on wavelength and these quantities will be different for the different frequency components of the pulse and will therefore be different for the pulse as a whole, compared

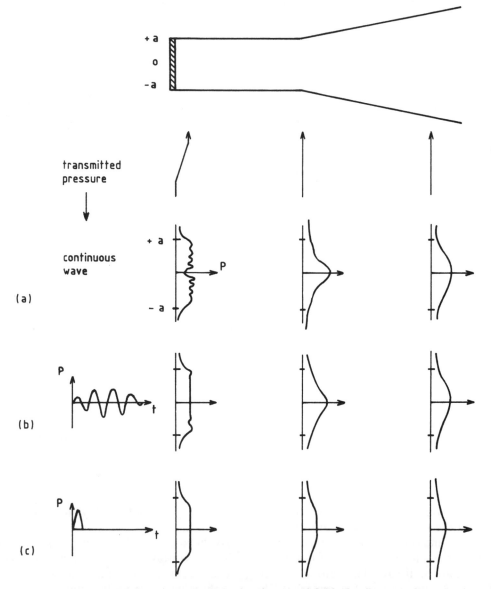

Figure 4.15 The variation in pressure at three points in the ultrasound field of a disc transducer for (a) continuous wave, (b) long pulse and (c) short pulse transmitted pressure waveforms. Adapted from Beaver W. L. (1974) Sonic nearfields of a pulsed piston radiator. *Journal of the Acoustical Society of America*, **56**, 1043–1048.

with the continuous wave of the same nominal frequency. Examples of pressure variation in the ultrasound field of a disc transducer for continuous wave, medium length and a short pulse are shown in Figure 4.15.

4.2.6 Beam Shape in Reception

We have considered the ultrasound field (beam) of the transducer used as a transmitter of ultrasound. It is also used as a receiver of reflected and backscattered ultrasound and we need to know the spatial variation of sensitivity or shape of the receiver beam.

By considering the total contribution over the transducer face of the ultrasound waves emanating from points in the ultrasound field, it is possible to show that the variation in sensitivity of the receiver beam has the same shape as the pressure variation in the field of the transducer used as a transmitter. The overall sensitivity—

being the variation of the received echo amplitude as a function of position in the beam—is given by the product of transmitted pressure and receiver beam sensitivity, and is thus proportional to the square of the transmitted pressure for a single transducer used as a transmitter and receiver. This is illustrated in Figure 4.16. Note that the net beam is narrower than the transmitted beam.

4.2.7 Transducer Selection

For different applications, we need to choose the transducer resonant frequency, diameter (aperture) and focal length. We do this by considering the requirements of penetration and resolution, and by using equation 4.2 and those in Figures 4.11 and 4.12. We will illustrate the selection process with two examples. Firstly consider a transducer for general abdominal scanning (Figure 4.17a).

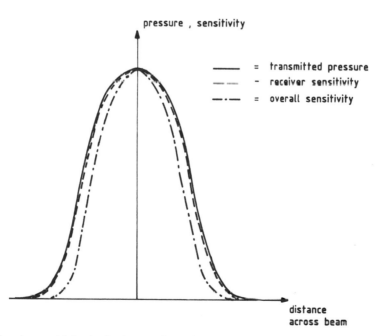

Figure 4.16 The variation in sensitivity in the beam of an ultrasound instrument (the variation in received signal from a small reflector with the position of the reflector) and its relationship to the variation in pressure in the transmitted beam and the variation in receiver sensitivity (received signal from a small source with the position of the source).

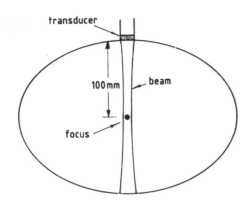

(a)

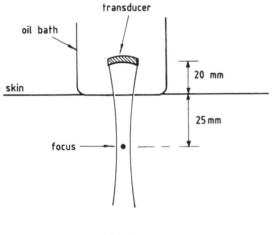

(b)

Figure 4.17 The transducer and beam shape required for (a) abdominal scanning and (b) superficial organ scanning.

Good resolution requires as high a frequency as possible. The penetration requirement limits this to 3.5 MHz. Therefore $f = 3.5$ MHz and from equation 2.2, using a value of $c = 1540$ m/s:

$$\lambda = 0.44 \text{ mm}$$

We wish to focus at mid-depth, and therefore we put:

$$R = 100 \text{ mm}$$

In order that the focal zone should have an adequate length we use weak focussing. Say:

$$Z_m/R = 2$$

giving (from equation 4.2)

$$Z_m = a^2/\lambda = 200 \text{ mm}$$

Substituting the value of λ gives:

$$a = 9.4 \text{ mm}$$

or a diameter ($2a$) of 18.8 mm.

The beam width at the focus (Figure 4.12) is:

$$d_f = \frac{R\lambda}{a} = 4.7 \text{ mm}$$

Secondly, consider a transducer for superficial organ scanning. The transducer is used in a mechanical real-time scanner where it is contained within an oil bath and offset by 20 mm from the skin surface (Figure 4.17b). This offset allows us to use medium focussing and a larger diameter transducer in order to obtain a narrower focus.

For superficial scanning we can use a frequency of 10 MHz. Therefore:

$$\lambda = 0.154 \text{ mm}$$

We wish to focus at 25 mm from the skin or 45 mm from the transducer. Therefore:

$$R = 45 \text{ mm}$$

For medium focussing we can use:

$$Z_m/R = 4$$

which gives

$$Z_m = a^2/\lambda = 180 \text{ mm}$$

and

$$a = 5.3 \text{ mm}$$

The beam width at the focus is:

$$d_f = \frac{R\lambda}{a} = 1.3 \text{ mm}$$

4.3 TRANSDUCERS

4.3.1 Piezoelectric Effect

Certain substances change their dimensions when an electric field is applied across them and conversely develop electrical charges on their surfaces when deformed. Such substances are called piezoelectric. The effect is called the piezoelectric effect. Examples of naturally occurring piezoelectric materials are quartz and lithium sulphate.

4.3.2 Transducer Material

If metallic electrodes are deposited on a thin plate of piezoelectric material, we can use such an arrangement as a transducer (Figure 4.18). It should be noted that the plate has to be cut in such a way that the molecules of the piezoelectric material are in a certain direction with respect to the cut of the plate. If the plate is compressed, then a potential difference will be detected across the silver electrodes and if the plate is stretched then the potential difference will reverse in sign (Figure 4.18a). It can therefore be used as a receiver of compressional waves. Conversely, if

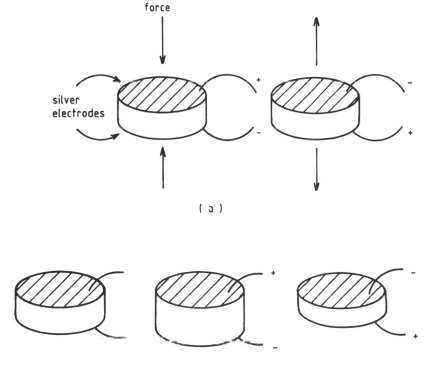

Figure 4.18 An electroded disc of piezoelectric material used as a receiver (a) and transmitter (b) of compressional waves.

a voltage is applied across the electrodes with one polarity, the plate will become thicker, and if the polarity is reversed, then the plate will become thinner (Figure 4.18b). It therefore has potential as a source or transmitter of compressional waves.

Obviously, for use as a transducer we want as efficient a conversion from electrical energy to mechanical energy and mechanical energy to electrical energy as possible and for this reason it is not usual to use naturally occurring piezoelectric materials, but rather artificial materials having a higher efficiency.

The most popular material for medical ultrasound transducers is known as PZT (lead zirconate titanate) which is not naturally piezoelectric but can be made so by poling (applying a high voltage across the electrodes whilst heating the material to a high temperature, causing the molecules in the material to line up in a preferred direction, and maintaining the high voltage while allowing to cool). The material, being a ceramic, is easily formed into suitable shapes for focussing.

4.3.3 Resonance

If a sinusoidal voltage is applied across a transducer, as shown in Figure 4.19, then continuous waves of ultrasound at the same frequency as the electrical signal are emitted from both surfaces. It is found that the amplitude of vibration of the surfaces peaks at certain frequencies.

Consider the situation illustrated in Figure 4.20.

The sinusoidal displacement of the transducer surface S_1 (Figure 4.20a) leads to the transmission of a displacement wave w_1 (Figure 4.20b). The surface movement also gives rise to a wave transmitted into the transducer itself which is partially reflected at surface S_2 and leads to a wave w_2 (Figure 4.20c) at surface S_1. If the thickness of the transducer (d) is chosen so that the transit time (τ) of the wave from S_1 to S_2 and back (distance = $2d$) is equal to the period of the oscillation, then waves w_1 and w_2 are in phase, they constructively interfere and the net displacement wave is as shown in Figure 4.20d. Clearly, there are other reflections within the

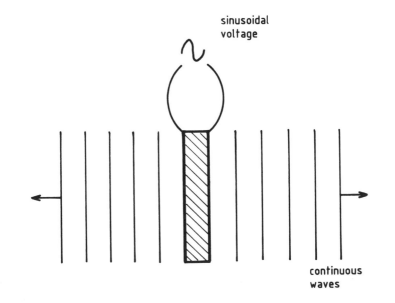

Figure 4.19 The continuous waves emitted from the front and rear surfaces of a transducer driven by a sinusoidal electrical signal.

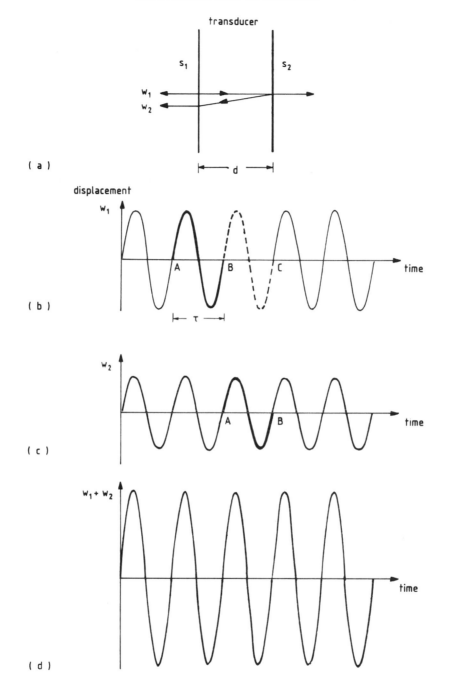

Figure 4.20 An illustration of resonance. The transducer and wave geometry (a), and the displacements of surface S_1 resulting from the initial displacement w_1 (b), the reflected wave w_2 (c) and the net displacement (d). The cycle AB in w_1 appears in the reflected wave w_2 after time τ. If this time delay is equal to the period of the ultrasound wave then AB in w_2 is coincident with the following cycle BC in the original displacement w_1 and the waves will constructively interfere to give a maximum net displacement w_1 plus w_2.

transducer leading to further enhancement of the transmitted wave. Note that this will also occur for waves from surface S_2.

Since waves travel one wavelength in the period of the wave, we have the condition for this to occur:

$$2d = \lambda_t$$

or   (4.3)

$$d = \lambda_t/2$$

where λ_t is the wavelength in the transducer material.

The frequency at which this occurs (the resonant frequency f_r) is given by:

$$f_r = c_t/\lambda_t$$
$$= c_t/(2d)$$ (4.4)

when c_t is the velocity of ultrasound in the transducer material.

If the frequency changes, then the waves w_1 and w_2 will no longer be in phase and the amplitude of the net transmitted wave will reduce. The transducer is said to resonate at frequency f_r.

Note that this resonant condition that waves w_1 and w_2 be in phase will also be satisfied if the reflected wave is delayed by a whole number of wavelengths (other than 1). A transducer will thus have other resonances at harmonics (integer multiples) of f_r. Increased losses in the transducer at high frequencies means that the transducer is less efficient (gives less mechanical power out for a given electrical power in) at these frequencies and medical transducers are always used at their fundamental resonant frequency.

The above description of resonance is equally true for mechanically or electrically induced vibration of the transducer surface and the transducer will thus resonate at the same frequency when used as a transmitter and as a receiver of ultrasound.

4.3.4 Pulsed Operation

For imaging purposes, we are interested in generating short pulses of ultrasound rather than continuous waves and this is achieved by applying very short voltage pulses across the transducer as shown in Figure 4.21. This causes the material to ring at the resonant frequency and the displacement of one of the faces (a damped sine wave) is shown. It should be noted that the movement of the surface is a very small fraction of the thickness of the transducer. The time taken for the ringing to die away (the pulse length) is determined by how much energy is lost during each half-cycle of oscillation. The energy is lost by attenuation in the transducer material itself and by transmission of energy into the media in contact with the front and rear faces of the transducer. We can reduce the pulse length by ensuring that as much energy as possible is lost from the rear surface of the transducer (the front surface being in contact with tissue). Since we know that the amount of ultrasound reflected at a boundary depends on the difference in acoustic impedance across the boundary, we can ensure loss of ultrasound into a backing material by making sure that its acoustic impedance is approximately the same as that of the transducer material. In addition, we need to make sure that the backing is absorbing, so that any ultrasound that gets into the backing material does not find its way back to the transducer. A suitable high-impedance, attenuating backing material can be made from loading epoxy resin with tungsten powder. Attenuation within the backing can be further increased by incorporating rubber powder. The backing is usually shaped as shown in Figure 4.22. The wedge shape ensures that multiple reflections of the ultrasound take place within the backing material, so increasing the path length and attenuation. The excess pressure waveforms following pulse excitation of the transducer are shown, for air-backing and high-impedance attenuating backing, in Figure 4.23.

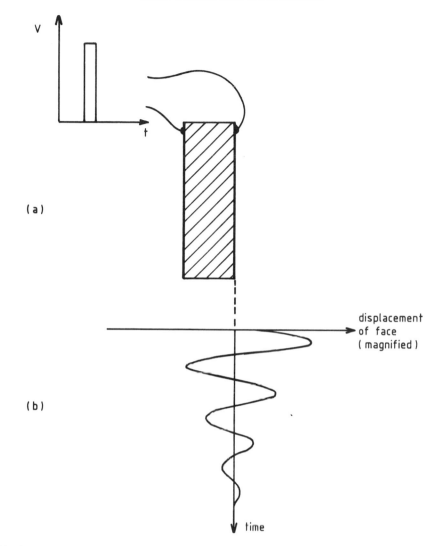

Figure 4.21 Ringing of a transducer following pulse excitation. Electrical pulse waveform and electrical connection (a), and surface displacement wave (b).

4.3.5 Matching Layer

At the front face of the transducer, we have the problem that the acoustic impedance of the transducer material is very much greater than the acoustic impedance of soft tissue. This means that the transmission of ultrasound from the transducer into the tissue is comparatively low. A method of improving this transmission is shown in Figure 4.24. A layer of material, one-quarter wavelength thick, of acoustic impedance between that of the transducer and tissue, is laid down on the transducer surface. A proportion of the ultrasound pressure pulse passing from the matching layer into the tissue is reflected back towards the transducer (reflection number 1). At interfaces where there is a drop in acoustic impedance there is a phase reversal during reflection and since Z_t is less than Z_m there is a phase reversal at this reflection. A proportion of this reflected

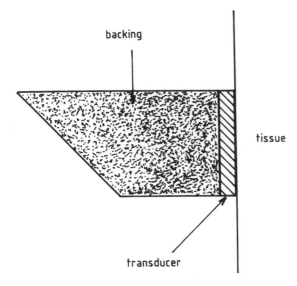

Figure 4.22 Backing for a pulsed transducer.

pulse is again reflected at the boundary between the transducer and the matching layer (reflection 2) and this twice-reflected pulse passes into the tissue. Since Z_x is greater than Z_m there is no phase reversal during reflection number 2. The twice-reflected pulse has travelled half a wavelength (two transits of one-quarter wavelength) and is reversed in polarity. When the first emitted pulse and the twice-reflected pulse are added together, it is noted that over part of the pulse length there is constructive interference and the net pulse amplitude is increased. There are subsequent reflections within the matching layer, giving rise to pulses of diminishing amplitude and all constructively interfering with the initial pulse.

It can be seen that making the layer on the transducer surface a quarter of a wavelength thick and with an impedance between that of the transducer and the tissue have led to an increase

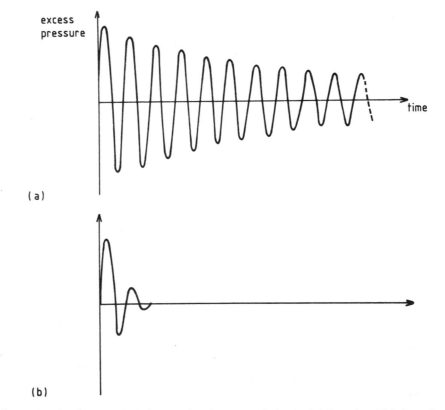

Figure 4.23 The transmitted excess pressure pulse from an air-backed (a) and a high-impedance-backed (b) transducer.

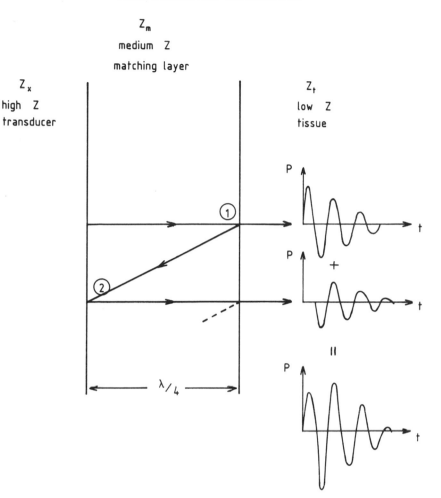

Figure 4.24 The quarter-wave matching layer.

in the emitted pulse amplitude. It is found that the acoustic impedance of the matching layer which gives rise to the maximum pulse height is the geometric mean of the transducer and tissue impedances:

$$Z_m = \sqrt{Z_x Z_t} \qquad (4.5)$$

For continuous wave ultrasound and assuming no attenuation within the matching layer, it can be shown, theoretically, that the transmission from transducer to tissue is 100%. In practice, the range of frequencies comprising a pulse means that the matching layer is not a quarter of a wavelength thick for all the frequency components and the transmission is somewhat less than 100% but still very much better than the situation with no matching layer. In order to improve still further the transducer efficiency over the bandwidth of short, imaging pulses, multiple matching layers may be used.

4.3.6 Probe Construction

The construction of unfocussed imaging (high-impedance-backed) and continuous wave (air-backed) transducers is shown in Figure 4.25. The

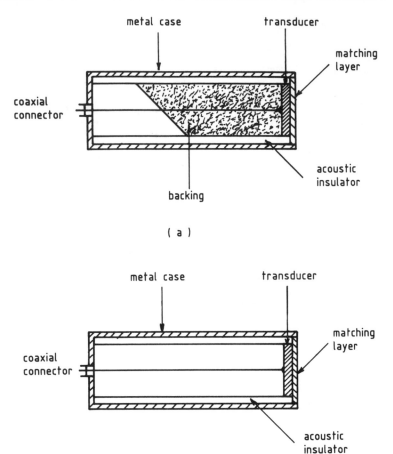

Figure 4.25 The construction of the pulsed (imaging) probe (a) and continuous wave (therapy) probe (b).

quarter-wave matching layer also provides some protection for the transducer crystal. The backing is enclosed within a metal case in order to provide a means of handling the transducer and to provide electrical shielding to prevent electrical interference being picked up when the transducer is being used as a receiver and to shield against the transmission of radio frequency electrical signals when the transducer is being used as a transmitter. An acoustic insulator (rubber or cork) is put between the transducer and the metal case to avoid transmission of ultrasound into the metal case. Electrical connections are made to the rear electrode on the transducer by the wire shown and to the front electrode via the metal case.

Note that sealing of the probe to prevent the ingress of moisture is important, not only to prevent damage to the probe, but also to maintain electrical insulation to avoid compromising electrical safety. Since probes may be damaged by heat, sterilising probes for interoperative use, for example, should be carried out using a sterilising liquid recommended by the manufacturer.

Focussed probes will have bowl-shaped transducers and matching layers as shown in Figure 4.26a. Since the concave front surface may trap bubbles in the jelly or oil used to acoustically

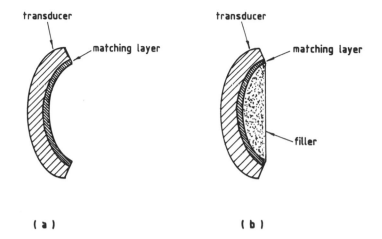

(a)   (b)

Figure 4.26 The focussed transducer with matching layer. Without filler (a) showing potential for bubble entrapment in the coupling jelly and with filler (b).

couple the probe to the skin surface, a flat-faced filler having a low acoustic impedance similar to that of tissue is often used (Figure 4.26b). Any refraction at the filler–tissue interface must be taken into account when calculating the transducer curvature to give the desired degree of focussing.

Note that we have considered here only single-element transducers. The double-element transducers used in continuous wave Doppler ultrasound and multi-element arrays used in real-time B-scanners will be described in the chapters dealing with these subjects.

CHAPTER 5

A-Scan Instruments

5.1 INTRODUCTION

Probably the simplest diagnostic ultrasound device is the A-scanner. A-scan instruments make use of the fact that the velocity of ultrasound in soft tissues is approximately constant (1540 m/s). This means that the time of flight of a pulse from the transducer to a reflector and back to the transducer can be used as a measure of the depth of the reflector. With reference to Figure 5.1 the delay time (τ) between transmission of an ultrasound pulse and the reception of the echo is:

$$\tau = 2L/c$$

or
$$L = \frac{c\tau}{2} \qquad (5.1)$$

and the depth of the reflector can be calculated from the time of arrival of the echo and knowledge of the velocity of propagation. In addition, the distance between reflectors can be calculated from the difference between the times of arrival of the echoes from the reflectors, as illustrated in Figure 5.2. That is:

$$L_1 = c\tau_1/2$$
$$L_2 = c\tau_2/2 \qquad (5.2)$$
$$D = L_2 - L_1 = \frac{c}{2}(\tau_1 - \tau_2)$$

Note that the use of a speed of ultrasound figure of 1540 m/s means that reflectors separated by 1 cm have echoes separated by 13 μs.

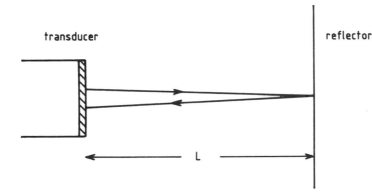

Figure 5.1 Pulse path between the transducer and reflector.

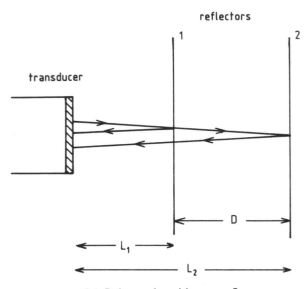

Figure 5.2 Pulse paths with two reflectors.

pulse. We can achieve this by using a cathode ray tube (CRT) display, connected as an oscilloscope (see Appendix D). The time base of an oscilloscope moves the spot on the screen across the screen at a fixed rate and the signal to be displayed, in this case the processed echo signal, appears as a vertical deflection of the spot. By starting the time base when the ultrasound pulse is transmitted, the echo signals are displayed at a position on the screen proportional to their time of arrival after transmission and this can be translated directly into a reading of the depth of the reflector, as shown in Figure 5.3.

5.3 INSTRUMENT DESIGN

The block diagram of a basic A-scan instrument is shown in Figure 5.4.

5.3.1 Master Clock and Transmitter

The part of the instrument which ensures that all the sections of the instrument function at the correct time is the PRF (pulse repetition

5.2 DISPLAY

A convenient way of displaying the depth of reflectors is to display the processed echo signals as a function of time following the transmitted

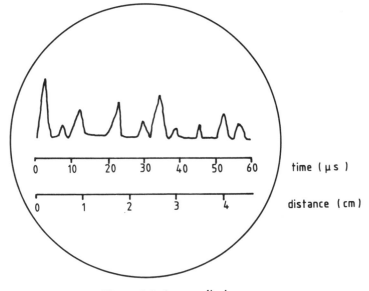

Figure 5.3 A-scan display.

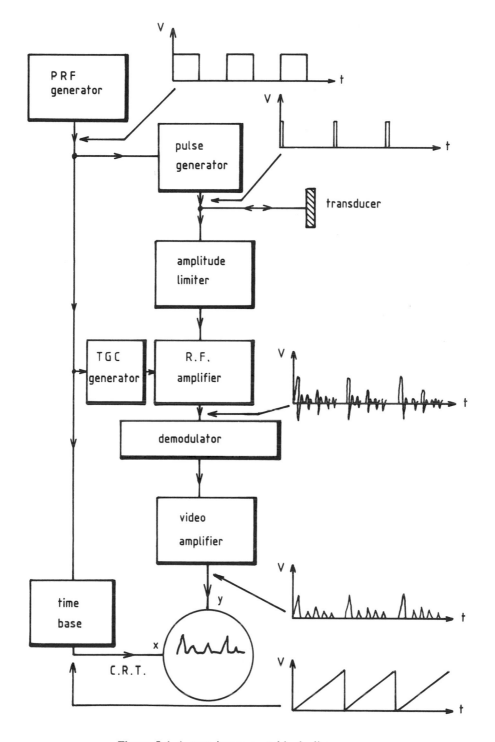

Figure 5.4 A-scan instrument block diagram.

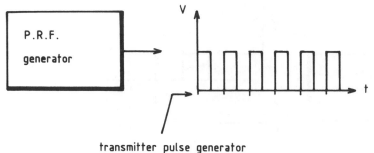

transmitter pulse generator
triggered at these times.

Figure 5.5 Output of the PRF generator or master clock.

frequency) generator—sometimes called the master clock. This is simply a generator of regularly spaced pulses as shown in Figure 5.5. On the leading edge of each clock pulse a short-pulse generator is triggered and this pulse is used to drive the transducer, which transmits a burst of ultrasound. At the same time, the time base for the oscilloscope display is started.

5.3.2 Receiver

Signals reflected from tissue interfaces are converted into electrical signals by the transducer and passed through an amplitude limiter to a radio frequency (RF) amplifier. The received signals are usually very much weaker than the transmitted signals since they have been attenuated in the tissue and reflected (in most cases) from weak reflectors. The amplifier increases the amplitude of these signals to useful levels. The amplitude limiter is required to protect the RF amplifier from the large-amplitude transmitted pulse.

5.3.3 Demodulator

The demodulator converts the short burst of radio frequency signal to a pulse for each reflector. The process is illustrated in Figure 5.6. The amplified received signal is passed to a rectifier, the output of which is filtered to remove

the higher frequency components, leaving a signal which is an approximation to the envelope of the received signal. Either a full-wave or half-wave rectifier can be used. A longer time constant for the filter following a half-wave rectifier is necessary to smooth out the individual half-cycles and this will result in a slightly longer pulse output, degrading the instrument's resolution slightly.

5.3.4 Display

The output from the demodulator is amplified in a video amplifier, the output of which is passed to the vertical deflection plates on the display CRT.

5.3.5 Time Gain Compensation (TGC)

As a result of attenuation of the ultrasound pulses, both in the path to a reflector and on the path back to the transducer, the echo signals from similar reflectors at different depths reduce in amplitude with depth as illustrated in Figure 5.7. We would like the displayed echo to be an indicator of reflector strength regardless of depth and in order to display echoes from similar reflectors at different depths at the same amplitude, we incorporate into the A-scan instrument a process of compensation for attenuation. This

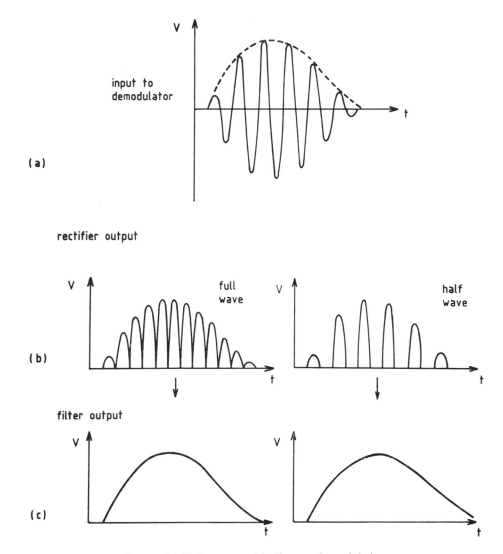

Figure 5.6 Full-wave and half-wave demodulation.

is achieved by increasing the gain of the RF amplifier with time, following each transmitted pulse, such that the increase in gain at a particular depth compensates for the attenuation of the signal from reflectors at that depth. This modification is shown in Figure 5.8. An RF amplifier with a voltage-controlled gain is used, such that an increase in the control voltage to the amplifier increases its gain. This control voltage is generated by a TGC (Time Gain Compensation) generator which is triggered by the PRF generator. Following each transmitted pulse, the TGC generator delivers an increasing voltage to the control voltage input of the RF amplifier, so increasing its gain with time following each transmitted pulse and thereby increasing the gain with depth of reflector. The display of the echoes from equal strength reflectors at different depths with the TGC switched off and switched on is shown in Figure 5.9.

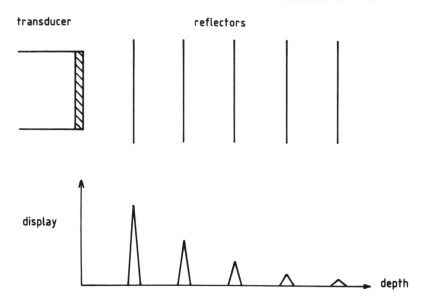

Figure 5.7 Demodulated echo pulses from similar reflectors in an attenuating medium.

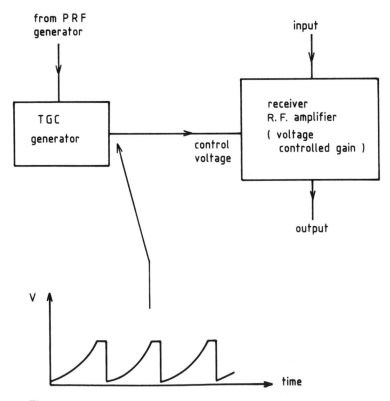

Figure 5.8 TGC block diagram and control voltage waveform.

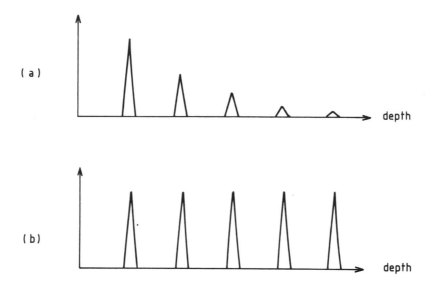

Figure 5.9 A-scan display with TGC off (a) and on (b).

One form for the shape of the TGC curve (which can often be displayed on the A-scan instrument) is shown in Figure 5.10a. Four controls can be used to alter the shape of this curve. The near gain is the gain to which echoes from close to the transducer are subjected. There is a variable delay before the increase of gain with depth. This delay can be set such that the gain is swept only over that range of depth which is of interest. The slope of the TGC curve can be altered to compensate for both high- and low-attenuation tissues and the maximum gain essentially limits the depth over which the gain is increased. A more flexible method of altering the TGC curve is illustrated in Figure 5.10b. In this case the gain at particular depths can be altered by using a number of gain controls distributed over the depth of interest. This allows for compensation for attenuation when the beam passes through tissues of different attenuation coefficients.

The TGC curve can be set automatically, as illustrated in Figure 5.11. The instrument averages the received echo strength and increases the gain with depth in order to keep the average displayed echo amplitude constant with depth.

5.4 DYNAMIC RANGE AND SIGNAL PROCESSING

5.4.1 Dynamic Range

There is a large range of received echo amplitudes from the very strong reflection at soft tissue–air interfaces to the scatter from small tissue structures, as shown in Table 5.1.

The dynamic range of signals (the range from the lowest level that can be detected—just above the noise—to the maximum signal level) at various points in the A-scan instrument is shown in Figure 5.12. It can be seen that it is necessary to reduce

Table 5.1 Echo amplitudes.

Reflecting/Scattering structure	Relative echo amplitude (dB)
Soft tissue–gas	0
Soft tissue–bone	−20
Fat–muscle	−40
Liver	−65
Brain	−100

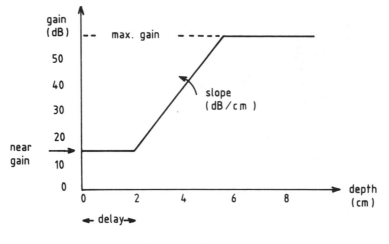

(a)

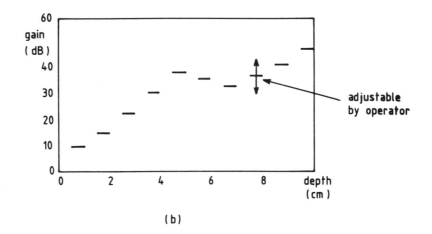

(b)

Figure 5.10 TGC curve (variation in receiver gain with depth). Single slope curve (a) and distributed gain control (b). Reproduced from McDicken, W.N. *Diagnostic Ultrasonics: Principles and Use of Instruments*, Churchill Livingstone, New York, 1981, with permission.

the large range of the received echoes in order to display them on the somewhat reduced range of the A-scan display.

5.4.2 Thresholding, Clipping and Windowing

Thresholding, as illustrated in Figure 5.13, can be used to display only those echoes which are above an operator-set threshold, in which case only the echoes from strong reflectors are displayed. Clipping (Figure 5.14) is used to limit the maximum amplitude of the signals sent to the display such that low-level echoes can be displayed without overloading the display. Windowing (dynamic range control) (Figure 5.15) is a combination of clipping and thresholding and

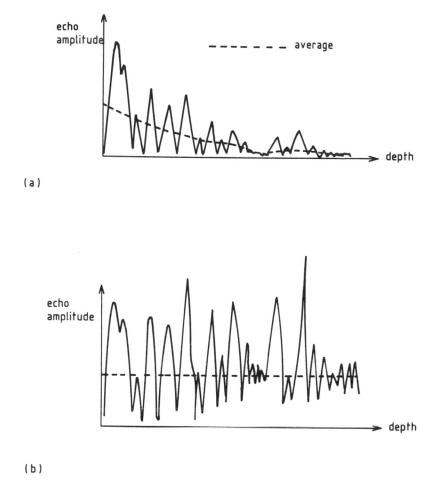

Figure 5.11 Automatic TGC showing running average with no TGC (a) and display with automatic gain control to give uniform running average (b). Adapted from McDicken, W.N. *Diagnostic Ultrasonics: Principles and Use of Instruments*, Churchill Livingstone, New York, 1981, with permission.

is used to select the range of echo amplitudes which are passed to the display.

5.4.3 Logarithmic Amplification

Logarithmic amplification as illustrated in Figure 5.16 is used, instead of a linear amplification of echo amplitudes, in order to selectively boost the level of low-level echoes, whilst compressing the range of high-level echoes. This allows the simultaneous display of echoes from the strongly reflecting organ boundaries with the weak echoes from the organ internal structure.

5.4.4 Differentiation and Edge Enhancement

Another form of signal processing used is differentiation, as illustrated in Figure 5.17. A differentiator has an output proportional to the rate of change of the input signal. It can be seen that this gives a short-duration pulse corresponding to the leading edge of an echo signal. The differentiator is used in the edge enhancement circuit, shown in Figure 5.18. The echo signal is passed to a differentiator and to a logarithmic amplifier and the outputs are added together,

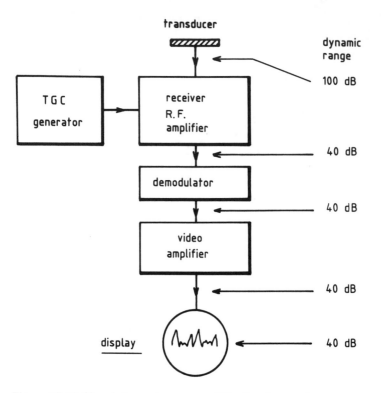

Figure 15.12 Signal dynamic ranges within the A-scan instrument.

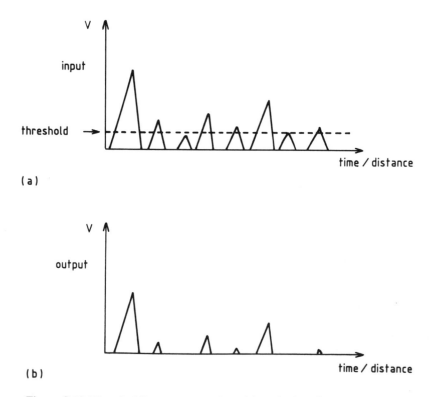

Figure 5.13 Thresholding. Signal before (a) and after (b) thresholding.

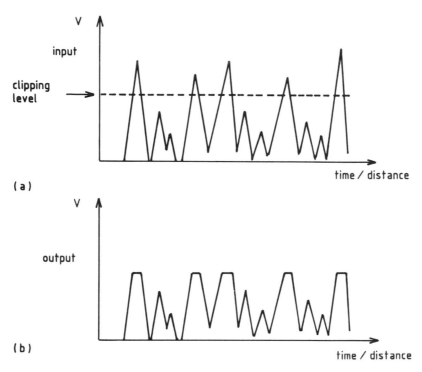

(a)

(b)

Figure 5.14 Clipping. Signal before (a) and after (b) clipping.

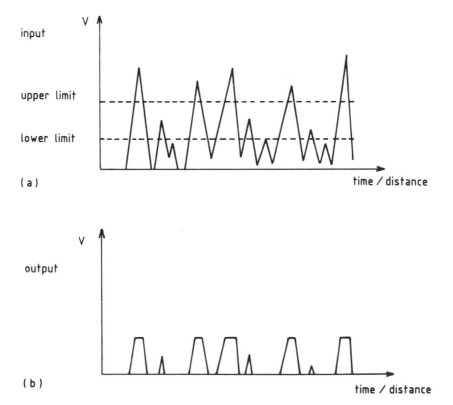

(a)

(b)

Figure 5.15 Windowing (dynamic range control). Signal before (a) and after (b) windowing.

62

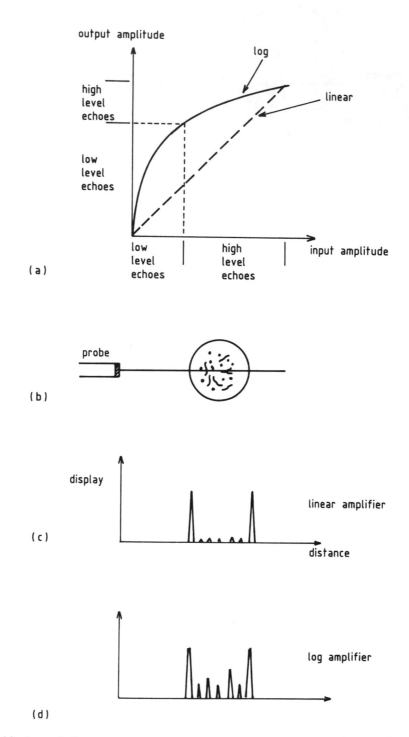

Figure 5.16 Logarithmic and linear gain receiver amplifiers. Transfer curves (a), probe/organ geometry (b), and display with linear (c) and logarithmic amplifiers (d).

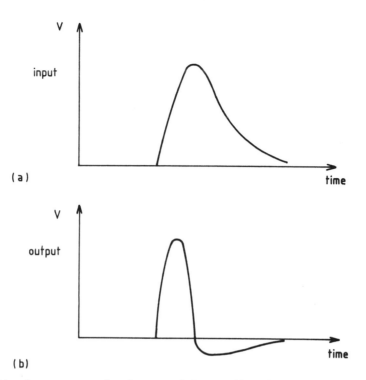

Figure 5.17 Differentiation (output proportional to rate of change of input). Input (a) and output (b) waveforms.

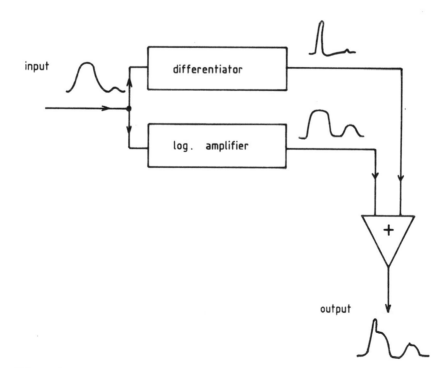

Figure 5.18 Edge enhancement. Block diagram of an edge enhancement circuit. Reproduced from McDicken, W.N. *Diagnostic Ultrasonics: Principles and Use of Instruments*, Churchill Livingstone, New York, 1981, with permission.

giving the signal illustrated. The proportions of the signals from the differentiator and from the logarithmic amplifiers are set such that there is a noticeable enhancement of the single large echoes from organ boundaries but no significant distortion of the image from the organ internal structure.

5.5 GAIN CONTROLS

The amplitude of the display signals can be changed by altering either the amplitude of the transmitted pulse or the gain of the receiver amplifier. The transmitted output control is often in the form of an attenuator, such that increasing attenuation will lead to a decrease in output. Increasing the output will lead to a proportionate increase in the level of all echoes. This is illustrated in Figure 5.19. Using the transmitter output control to increase the displayed echo amplitude has the disadvantage that it increases patient dose. Alternatively, the amplitude of the displayed echoes can be increased by increasing the receiver amplifier gain. The disadvantage of this method is that at high gain, noise generated within the receiver amplifier will be displayed. This is illustrated in Figure 5.20.

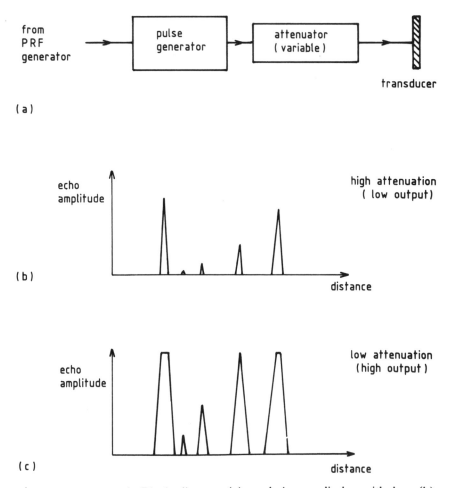

Figure 5.19 Transmitter output control. Block diagram (a), and A-scan display with low (b) and high (c) transmitter output.

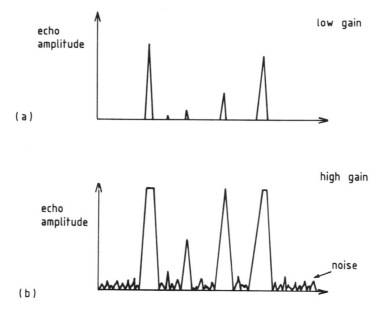

Figure 5.20 Receiver amplifier gain. The display with low (a) and high (b) receiver amplifier gain.

5.6 PENETRATION

Since the amplitude of the echoes decreases (through attenuation) with depth and since increasing the receiver gain increases the level of the displayed electronic noise, there comes a point where, for maximum transmitted output, the echo signals are masked by the noise. The depth at which echoes are just distinguishable above the background noise is known as the depth of penetration.

5.7 AXIAL RESOLUTION

Axial resolution is a measure of the instrument's ability to separate the echoes from reflectors which are closely spaced along the ultrasound beam axis. The distance between reflectors which are just resolved is a measure of resolution.

Resolution is often illustrated by considering the overlap and addition of the contributions of two displayed (demodulated) echoes. In practice, the overlapping parts of each echo combine at the transducer and lead to interference effects. An illustration of the received and displayed echoes from two reflectors at four different separations is given in Figure 5.21.

As a result of the slope on the rising and falling edges of the displayed echo from a reflector, increasing the overall gain, either by increasing the transmitter output or the receiver amplifier gain, will increase the length of the displayed echo, as illustrated in Figure 5.22. The increase in echo amplitude combined with clipping or high-amplitude compression can lead to a decrease in the ability to resolve the echoes from close reflectors.

5.8 PULSE REPETITION FREQUENCY (PRF)

The transducer is pulsed periodically so that the operator can see the display changing as the orientation of the ultrasound beam is adjusted in order to arrive at the optimum orientation—

reflector separation   receiver signal   display

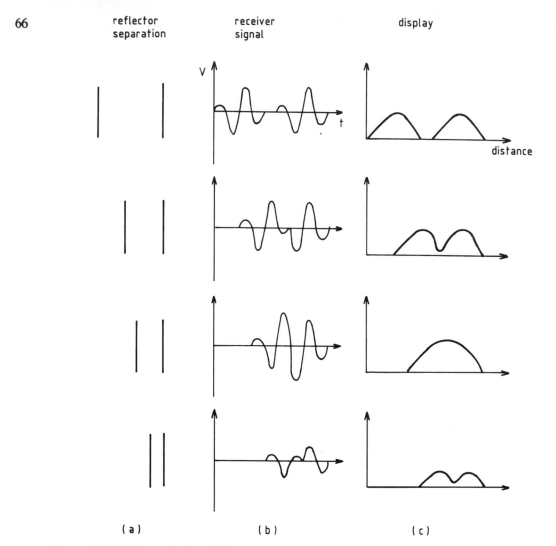

Figure 5.21 Axial resolution. Reflector separation (a), received signal (b) and A-scan display (c).

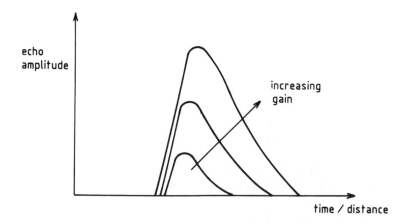

Figure 5.22 The effect of gain on the displayed echo.

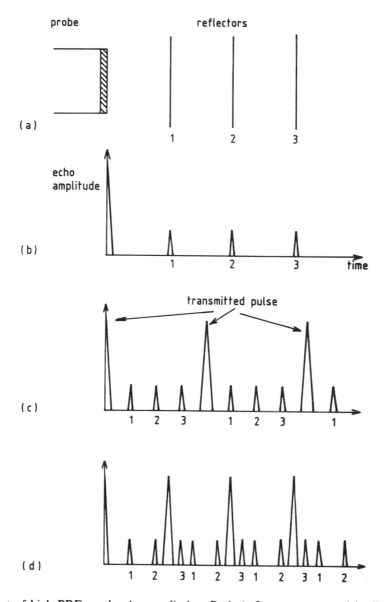

Figure 5.23 The effect of high PRF on the A-scan display. Probe/reflector geometry (a), display with low PRF (b) and with compressed timescale (c) and the display with too high a PRF (d).

passing through the tissues of interest. There is a limitation on the PRF, as illustrated in Figure 5.23. Graph (b) shows the normal display of echoes received from reflectors, numbered 1–3. Graph (c) shows the signal with a slower time base, showing a number of consecutive

transmission–reception sequences. If the time between each transmitted pulse is reduced (an increase in PRF) then the next transmitted pulse is emitted before the reception of the most distant echo (graph (d)). In this case the display of the echoes would be in the incorrect order (3,1,2).

It is clear that the time between transmission pulses must be greater than the transit time of the transmitted pulse to the maximum depth of penetration and back to the transducer. This leads to the constraint on the pulse repetition period and pulse repetition frequency as shown below:

$$\text{Minimum pulse repetition period } (T_\text{p}) = \frac{2L_{\max}}{c}$$

$$\text{or} \qquad \text{Maximum PRF} = \frac{c}{2L_{\max}} \qquad (5.3)$$

where $L_{\max}$ = maximum depth of penetration.

CHAPTER 6

Static B-Scan

6.1 INTRODUCTION

The A-scanner gives information on the position of reflectors/scatterers along the ultrasound beam. By sensing the position and orientation of the beam this information, together with the depth (along the beam), can be used to calculate the position of echo-generating structures and indicate their position on a screen (Figure 6.1). If the beam is moved, while confined to a plane (scan plane), an image of echo-generating structures cut by the plane can be built up as shown in Figure 6.2.

The static B-scanner, in which the beam is moved by manually moving a single transducer, has (almost entirely) been replaced by the real-time scanner (Chapter 7). Nevertheless, it is

worth a brief mention since it provides a useful introduction to B-scanning in general.

6.2 THE CRT DISPLAY

6.2.1 Display Drive Signals

A cathode ray tube (CRT) can be used as the image display device, as shown in Figure 6.3. Voltage ramps are applied to the x (horizontal) and y (vertical) deflection plates in order to move the electron beam-generated spot across the screen, along a line corresponding to the ultrasound beam, at a speed corresponding to 13 μs/cm in tissue. The ramps (time bases) are started (triggered) at the same time as the transmitter

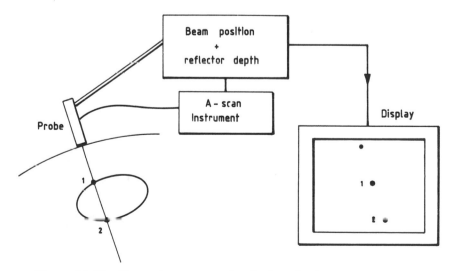

Figure 6.1 The B-scan instrument—the display of echoes as bright spots.

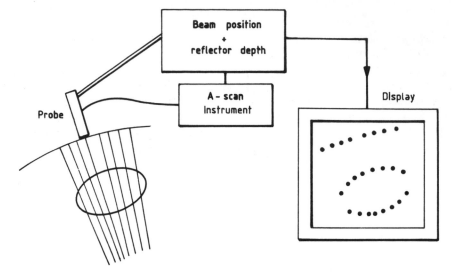

Figure 6.2 The generation of a B-scan display.

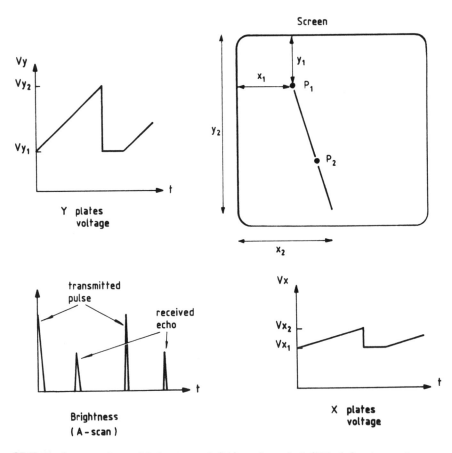

Figure 6.3 The CRT display together with horizontal (V_x) and vertical (V_y) deflection voltages and brightness modulation. P_1 indicates the position of the transducer and the spot is generated by the transmitter pulse. P_2 is the echo from a single reflector.

pulse is emitted. The starting voltages (V_{x1}, V_{y1}) give a spot position corresponding to the probe face. The spot reaches a position corresponding to the position of a reflector at the same time as the echo from that reflector is received, and the A-scan signal is used to modulate the electron beam in the CRT so that the spot is brightened by the echo signals.

6.2.2 Bistable and Greyscale Display

The display can be bistable, in which case an echo is displayed on the screen if the echo signal is above a pre-set threshold, or greyscale, in which case the brightness of the echo display is governed by the amplitude of the echo (Figure 6.4). Bistable systems are generally only suitable

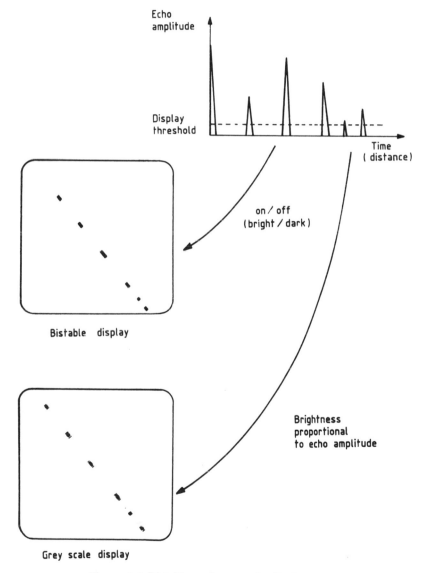

Figure 6.4 Bistable and greyscale displays.

for showing strong reflectors, such as organ boundaries. Greyscale displays can also show the weaker scattered signals from organ parenchyma.

6.2.3 Persistence

The image brightness will decrease with time after being 'written' on the screen. The rate of decrease is governed by the phosphor on the CRT screen and the display is specified by its 'persistence', which refers to the length of time the image remains visible on the screen after being written (Figure 6.5). Long-persistence screens have the advantage that the image may be viewed for longer, but shorter persistence is required when it is necessary to follow movement of echoes.

6.2.4 Display Co-ordinate Signal Generation

As shown in Figure 6.6, the spot deflection signals to the CRT are generated by combining x and y time base ramps together with signals from a probe position and orientation sesnsors to which the probe is mechanically coupled.

6.3 PROBE POSITION AND ORIENTATION SENSING

6.3.1 Co-ordinate Systems

The position of points in a plane can be specified by two different co-ordinate systems—Cartesian (Figure 6.7a), requiring the distances x and y from perpendicular axes, and polar (Figure 6.7b), requiring the distance r from an origin point and the angle (θ) between the line joining the point to the origin and the reference line.

6.3.2 Mechanical Systems

There are two main methods of probe position and orientation sensing, as shown in Figure 6.8. In the gantry arrangement (Figure 6.8a) the probe can rotate on a movable pivot, the Cartesian co-ordinates of which are given by potentiometers connected to sense the linear movements shown.

The signals from the gantry are those from the potentiometers sensing the Cartesian co-ordinates of the pivot and from a potentiometer sensing the angle (θ) of the rotation of the probe. In the articulated arm arrangement (Figure 6.8b) the

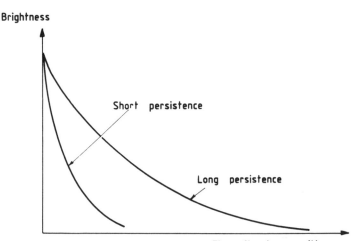

Figure 6.5 Screen phosphor persistence.

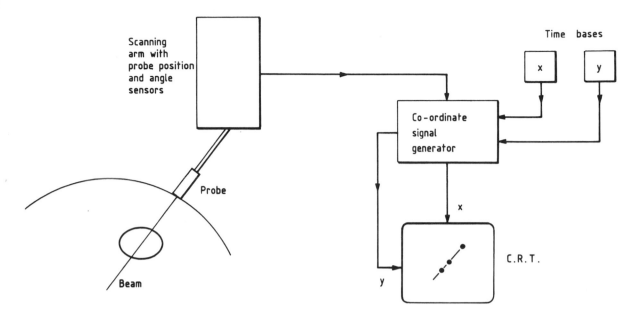

Figure 6.6 Display co-ordinate generation.

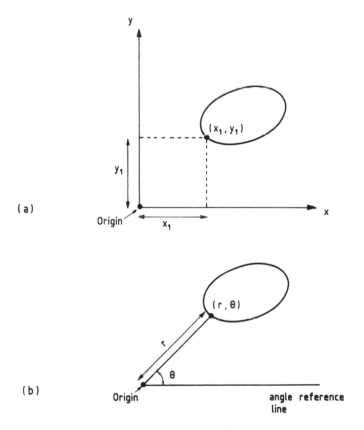

Figure 6.7 Cartesian (a) and polar (b) co-ordinate systems.

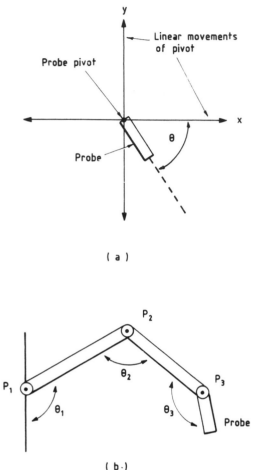

(a)

(b·)

Figure 6.8 Probe position and orientation sensing. Gantry (a) and articulated arm (b).

probe is connected via two articulated arms to a stationary pivot P1. Potentiometers sense the angles θ_1, θ_2 and θ_3 and these, together with the arm lengths, are used to calculate the position and orientation of the probe.

6.4 B-SCANNER BLOCK DIAGRAM

A block diagram of the manual B-scanner is shown in Figure 6.9. It consists of an A-scan instrument in conjunction with a probe position and orientation-sensing mechanism, a display co-ordinate signal generator and a (CRT) display.

6.5 THE SCAN CONVERTER

An alternative and more usual display is a video monitor on which the spot on the screen is repetitively moved in a raster fashion as shown in Figure 6.10 (see also Appendix D). In this case, a scan converter takes in image information in the scan format of the B-scanner and puts out the same image in the raster format (Figure 6.11). The scan converter will be examined in more detail later on. The B-scan instrument now has the form shown in Figure 6.12.

6.6 SCANNING PATTERNS

The operator is free to adopt a number of different scan patterns and in order to appreciate the effect on the image of each method, it is necessary to re-examine the mechanism of echo generation. As indicated in Figure 6.13, a specular reflector will give rise to a large echo when it is perpendicular to the beam since pulses are reflected straight back to the probe. However, the reflector has to be at only a small angle to this ideal orientation with respect to the beam for the reflected pulse to miss the transducer completely. Thus the strength of the echo from a specular reflector is large and at a maximum for perpendicular incidence of the beam, but reduces rapidly with angle. On the other hand, scatter from a rough surface, or from small structures, covers a wide range of angles and the orientation of the probe is much less critical. The most common simple scans (in which the beam passes through each point in the scan plane only once) are linear and sector (Figure 6.14a). A compound scan in which the beam passes through points in the scan plane from more than one direction during the scan is shown in Figure 6.14b.

As a result of limited beam/reflector angle tolerance, when imaging specular reflectors, only a small part of an organ boundary, perpendicular or close to perpendicular to the beam direction, is imaged when a simple scan pattern is used (Figure 6.15a). A greater proportion of the

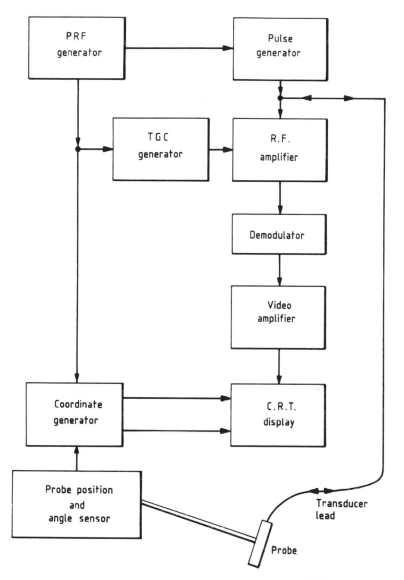

Figure 6.9 Block diagram of B-scan instrument with CRT display.

boundary is perpendicular to a beam direction at some time during the scan when a compound scanning pattern is used (Fig. 6.15b). The disadvantage is that the compound scan takes longer and there is more chance of image distortion due to patient (e.g. fetal) movements during the scan.

6.7 WATER BATH SCANNING

A water bath (Figure 6.16) is sometimes used for scanning in order to remove the probe from contact with the skin surface. There are two reasons for this. Firstly, superficial tissues can

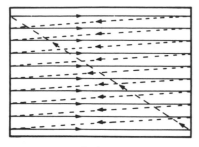

(a)

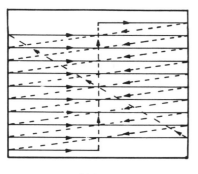

(b)

Figure 6.10 Video monitor raster. Simple (a) and interlaced (b).

be distorted by the scanning movement, since pressure is required to maintain contact free from air bubbles during contact scanning. The water bath eliminates this problem. Secondly, as illustrated in Figure 6.17, the electrical signal resulting from the 'ringing' of the transducer following the transmitter drive pulse is larger than that of, and will swamp received echoes from, reflectors close to the transducer. This ringing leads to a dead zone, close to the transducer, in which tissues cannot be imaged. Removing the transducer from the skin surface using a water bath removes this problem.

An automated water bath scanner is shown in Figure 6.18. The patient lies prone on top of the water bath in which eight focussed transducers each perform a sector scan—the combination giving a compound scan.

6.8 RESOLUTION

As in the A-scan instrument the axial resolution—the ability to separate images from reflectors which are close along the direction of the beam—is governed primarily by the transmitter pulse length. The lateral resolution is governed by beam width. The instrument will show the echo of a structure within the beam as if it were on the beam axis. Figure 6.19 illustrates how the width of the image of a reflector is increased by the width of the beam.

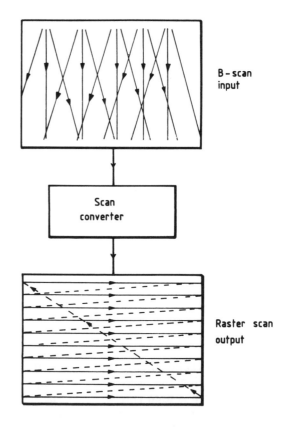

B-scan input

Scan converter

Raster scan output

Figure 6.11 Scan converter input and output scan patterns.

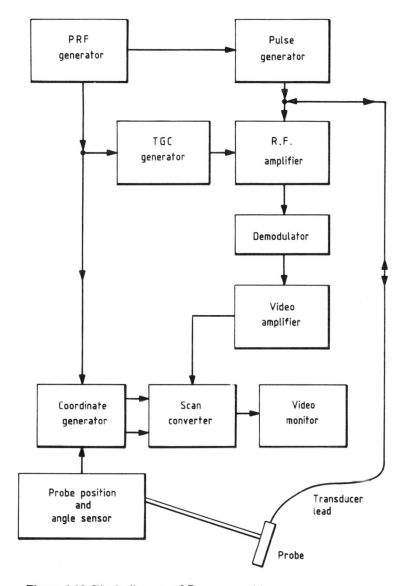

Figure 6.12 Block diagram of B-scanner with scan converter.

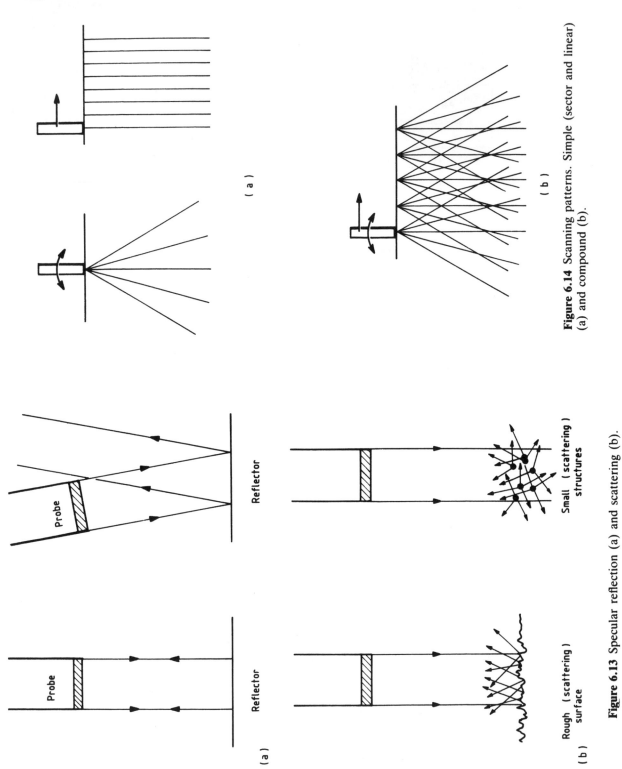

Figure 6.14 Scanning patterns. Simple (sector and linear) (a) and compound (b).

Reflector

Probe

Reflector

Small (scattering) structures

Rough (scattering) surface

Figure 6.13 Specular reflection (a) and scattering (b).

(a)

(b)

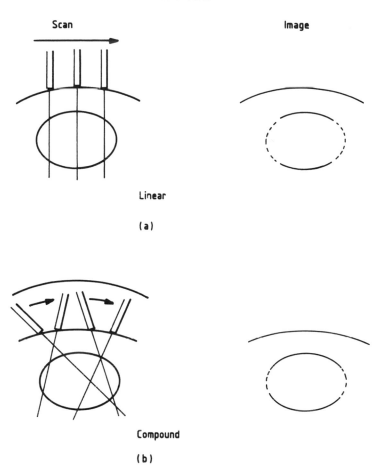

Figure 6.15 Organ boundary image with simple linear scan (a) and compound scan (b).

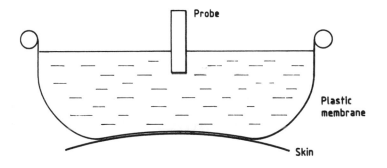

Figure 6.16 Water bath scanning.

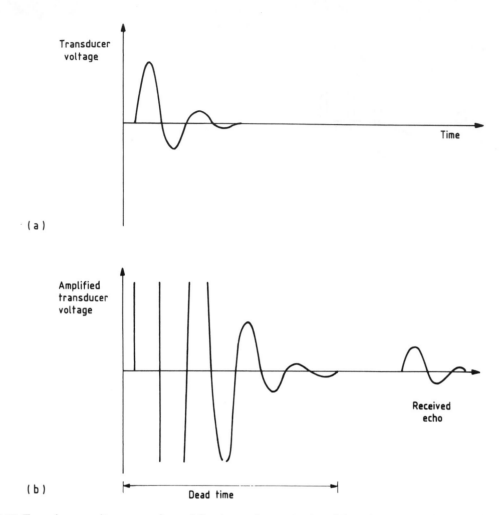

Figure 6.17 Transducer voltage waveform following pulse excitation (a) and corresponding receiver amplifier output (b) indicating instrument dead time.

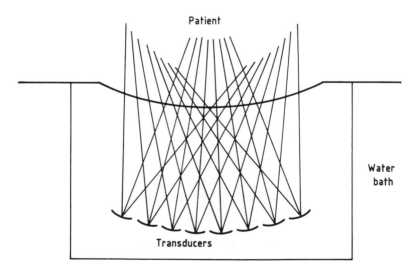

Figure 6.18 An automated water bath scanner.

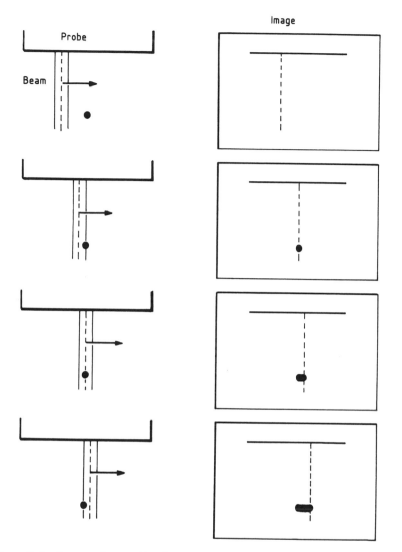

Figure 6.19 Formation of the image of a small reflector during a linear scan showing the effect of beam width.

CHAPTER 7

Real-time Scanners

7.1 INTRODUCTION

Real-time scanners were developed in order to monitor moving structures (heart, fetus) and to provide nearly instantaneous response to a change of scan plane. In such scanners the ultrasound beam is swept automatically and repetitively through the scan plane usually at such a rate that the image appears free from flicker. The beam can be swept mechanically or electrically and we shall consider the different types in turn.

7.2 MECHANICAL SCANNERS

The types of mechanical scanner probes are shown in Figure 7.1. In all cases, the ultrasound transducer is within an oil bath with a thin rubber/plastic membrane 'window' through which the ultrasound beam passes. The movement necessary to sweep the beam is provided by a motor.

The probe may be moved in a rectilinear fashion (Figure 7.1a), the probe may be fixed and the beam reflected by an oscillating mirror (Figure 7.1b), the probe itself may be rocked backwards and forwards (Figure 7.1c) or three or four transducers may be mounted on the periphery of a rotating wheel (Figure 7.1d). In the latter case, switches ensure that a transducer is active only when its beam can pass through the window. The scan plane is rectangular in Figure 7.1a and sector shaped in the rest. The most common types are shown in Figures 7.1c

and d. To avoid large refraction errors and large reflections at the window, the characteristic velocities and impedances of the oil and window material are usually chosen to be close to those of soft tissue.

7.2.1 Instrument Block Diagram

The block diagram of a mechanical real-time scanner, based on a rotating wheel probe, is shown in Figure 7.2. Most of the instrument is the same as a static B-scan instrument. However, in this case the scan converter obtains beam orientation information from a position encoder coupled to the wheel drive shaft. The electrical connections to the transducers must be taken in via bushes and slip rings, or a particular type of transformer in which primary and secondary windings are free to rotate with respect to each other. Each of the transducers on the wheel has the same associated components as a static B-scan probe. They are: electrical connections to the transducer which is focussed by shaping or by a lens, a matching layer, high impedance, strongly absorbing backing and electrical screening.

The rocking transducer and rocking mirror real-time scanners are very similar, with an encoder sensing probe or mirror position. Slip rings are not necessary in this case since there is no continuous rotation of the probe.

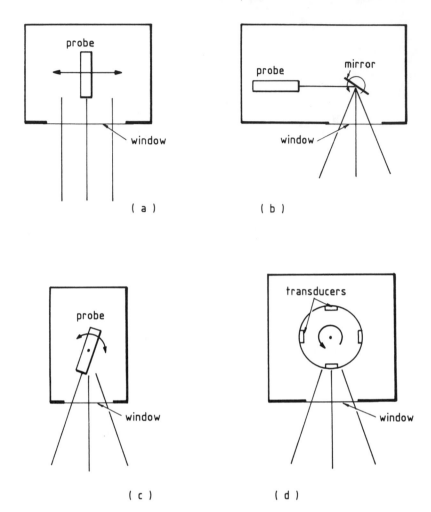

Figure 7.1 Mechanical scanner probes. Rectilinear movement (a), rocking mirror (b), oscillating probe (c) and rotating wheel (d).

7.3 THE ANNULAR ARRAY AND ELECTRONIC FOCUSSING

The transducers in mechanical real-time scanners sometimes employ electronic focussing. The transducers employed are split into a number of concentric annuli as shown in Figure 7.3. Their focussing action is illustrated in Figure 7.4, where the annular array elements are shown in section along the diameter of a transducer.

7.3.1 Focussing in Transmission

In order to achieve focussing during transmission (Figure 7.4a), delays are introduced in the excitation pulse to each element of the array. If the delays are arranged as shown such that there is a greater delay in the application of the pulse to, and therefore in the transmission of the pulse from, the centre element, then the part of the wavefront from the outer annulus will have

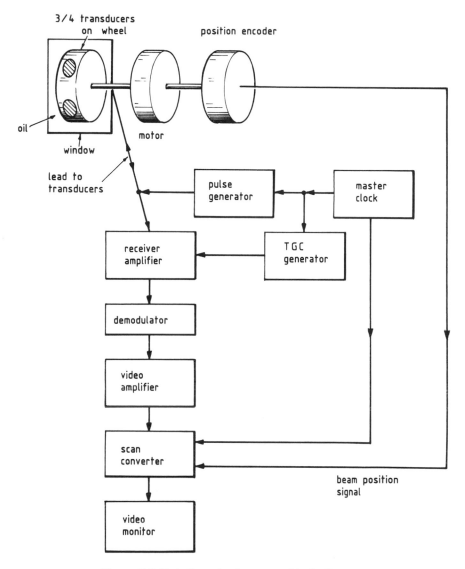

Figure 7.2 Rotating wheel scanner block diagram.

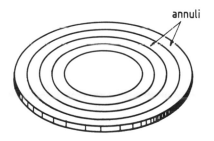

Figure 7.3 The annular array.

travelled a greater distance at any instant than that from the centre, the wavefront will have the concave shape shown and the wave will converge to a focus.

The position of the focus can be changed by altering the delays in order to change the curvature of the emitted wavefront. The closer the focus, the greater the curvature of the wavefront and the greater the difference in delay between centre and outer annuli.

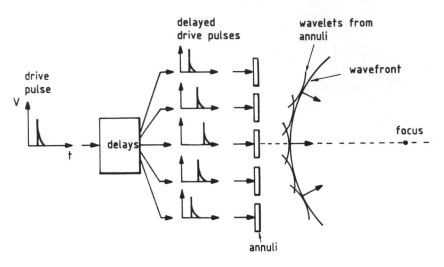

(a)

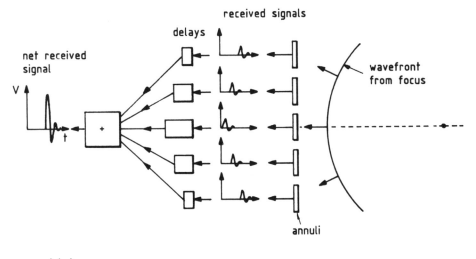

(b)

Figure 7.4 Electronic focussing in transmission (a) and reception (b). Note that the drive pulses and received signals are shown plotted against time whereas the wavefronts are shown as a 'snapshot' view.

An alternative view of the focussing mechanism is that the focus is the point at which the pulses from all the annuli arrive simultaneously. Thus, the focus is the point for which the sum of electronic delay and pulse transit time through the tissue to the point is the same for each annulus.

7.3.2 Focussing in Reception

To achieve focussing in reception (Figure 7.4b) the received signal from each annulus is delayed before adding. Again, there is a focus at a point when the transit time of the echo pulse from the point plus the electronic delay is the same for each annulus. As for transmission, this requires a greater delay for the centre of the transducer than for the outside and the focus can be brought closer to the transducer by increasing the difference between the delays.

Note that the transducer is axially symmetric and the same degree of focussing is achieved across any beam diameter at a particular distance from the transducer.

7.3.3 Circuit for Electronic Focussing

A block diagram of the circuit required for transmission focussing is shown in Figure 7.5. Each annulus has its own high-voltage pulse generator, since the controllable delays operate at low voltage. The circuit required for receiver beam focussing is shown in Figure 7.6. Preamplifiers are used to boost the level of the signal

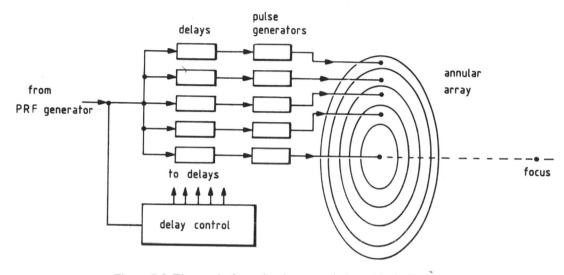

Figure 7.5 Electronic focussing in transmission—block diagram.

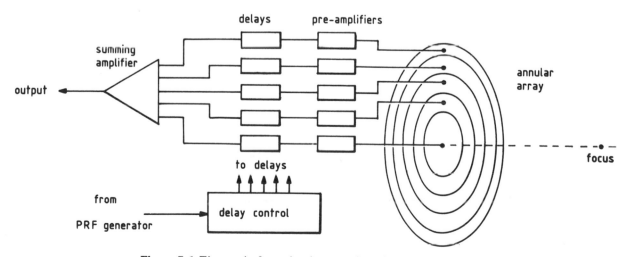

Figure 7.6 Electronic focussing in reception—block diagram.

from each annulus before it is passed to the delay, since this is a point at which noise can enter the signal path.

7.3.4 Multiple Zone Focussing (Transmission)

The transmitted beams can be focussed at different depths by altering the delays leading, for example, to the beam shapes labelled 1–4 in Figure 7.7. All these beam shapes can be used together in a mode of operation called multiple zone focussing. In this mode, at any one beam orientation, the instrument uses focus 1 and displays echoes returned from the focal zone of this beam. It then switches to focus 2 and displays echoes from the focal zone of this beam and so on with beams 3 and 4. The equivalent beam shape is that shown as a dashed line. It should be noted that since the echoes for each focus have to return before changing the focus and transmitting the next pulse in order to avoid mis-registration of echoes, the frame rate for the multiply focussed beams is reduced by a factor $1/N_z$ where N_z is the number of focal zones.

7.3.5 Dynamic Focussing (Reception)

The focus can also be altered during the scan in reception. In this case, however, the focus can be altered during the reception of echoes from each transmitted pulse and is called dynamic focussing. The receiver delays are switched to give a focus, close to the transducer following transmission and switched to the next focus when the received echoes move from the first to the second focal zone. This continues for the other foci. There is no PRF reduction penalty for dynamic focussing. The equivalent beam shape for reception is similar to that for multiple zone focussing.

7.3.6 Scanner Circuit Modifications

Focussing in transmission and reception are usually both available, and a mechanical B-scan instrument incorporating these facilities has the additional features shown in Figure 7.8.

7.3.7 Apodisation and Dynamic Aperture Control

As we have seen in Chapter 4, while most of the emitted ultrasound power is concentrated in one lobe, there can be some 'leakage' of power into side lobes (also present in the receiver beam) and the presence of these lobes can lead to spurious echo registration. The intensity of these

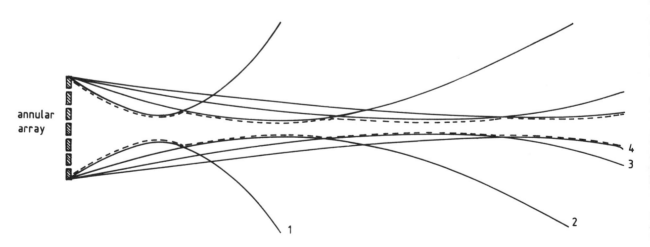

Figure 7.7 Multiple zone focussing.

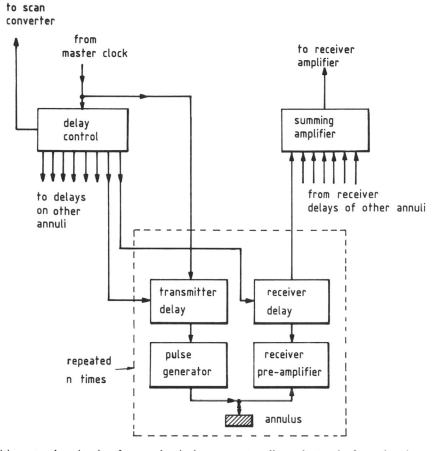

to scan
converter

from
master clock

to receiver
amplifier

delay
control

summing
amplifier

to delays
on other
annuli

from receiver
delays of other annuli

transmitter
delay

receiver
delay

repeated
n times

pulse
generator

receiver
pre-amplifier

annulus

Figure 7.8 Additions to the circuit of a mechanical scanner to allow electronic focussing in transmission and reception.

side lobes can be reduced by apodisation—reducing the amplitude of vibration of the transducer towards the edge of the transducer in the transmitter mode and the sensitivity towards the edge in the receive mode. This is easily achieved with an annular transducer by simply altering the amplitude of the transmitted drive pulse to the annuli and the gain of the receiver preamplifiers. The degree of apodisation can be altered to suit the different side lobe suppression requirements at different degrees of focussing.

The beam shape can be improved still further by dynamic aperture control, switching out the outer annuli when the focal length is small in order to achieve a longer focal zone (Figure 7.9).

7.4 THE LINEAR ARRAY

7.4.1 Construction and Operation

The probe of this device consists of a linear array of small transducer elements (Figure 7.10). A group of neighbouring elements are used together to form a transducer which projects a beam as shown. The beam is moved by moving the group forming the transducer by one element at a time for successive transmission pulses. This process is shown in Figure 7.11.

A block diagram of a real-time scanner using a linear array is shown in Figure 7.12. Again, most of the elements of the instrument are those

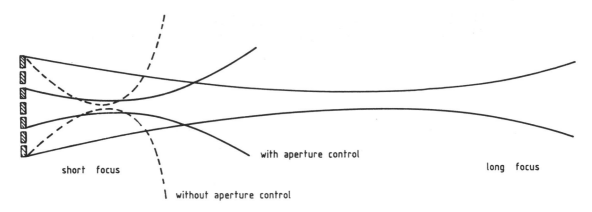

short focus

with aperture control

without aperture control

long focus

Figure 7.9 Dynamic aperture control.

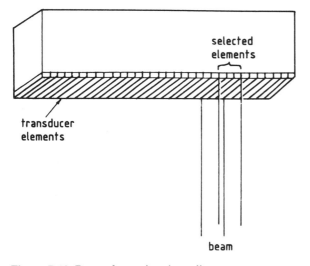

selected elements

transducer elements

beam

Figure 7.10 Beam formation in a linear array transducer.

found in a static B-scanner. The instrument has electronic switches which are used to select the elements for each beam and the switches are activated in the required sequence by an element-switching-logic circuit driven by the master clock.

The scan converter receives timing information from the master clock to enable the depth of reflectors to be registered and a beam position signal from the element switching logic.

7.4.2 Focussing

The beam can be focussed in transmission and reception in the same fashion as an annular array (simply read 'elements' for 'annuli' in the description) and the same circuit modification is required. This electronic focussing, however, takes place only in the scan plane. There is no focussing action to reduce the width of the scan plane (slice thickness) as there is with the annular array. Fixed focussing, using shaped elements or a cylindrical lens (Figure 7.13), can be used to reduce slice thickness. Dynamic aperture control to improve focal zone length close to the transducer and apodisation to reduce side lobe levels can be used as with the annular array.

7.4.3 The Curvilinear Array

One of the advantages of the rectangular scan of the linear array scanner compared with the sector scan of the common types of mechanical scanner is the width of the scan close to the skin. The accompanying disadvantage is that a large area of skin contact is required. An arrangement giving a scan field somewhere between the extremes of the sector and rectangular scans is the curvilinear array (Figure 7.14). Such a probe

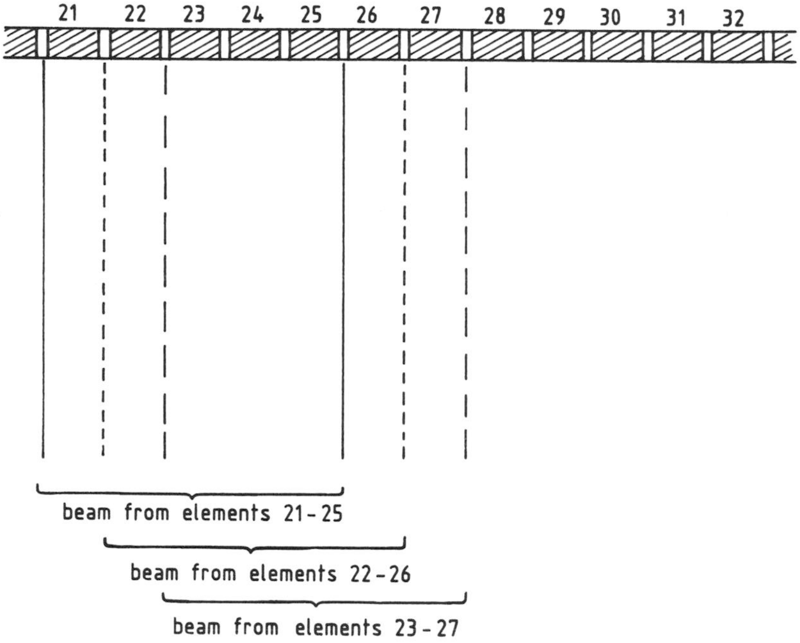

Figure 7.11 Linear array beam movement.

operates in a similar way to a linear array probe. The convex shape, however, gives a larger field of view at a given depth than for a linear array having the same contact area.

7.5 THE PHASED ARRAY SCANNER

7.5.1 Construction and Operation

A sector scan can be produced without moving parts using a phased array scanner, the probe of which is shown in Figure 7.15. This consists of a small array of transducer elements and the beam steering is achieved by means of variable electronic delays connected to each element as used in the focussing of annular arrays. The mechanism of electronic beam steering is illustrated in Figure 7.16a. The principle is very similar to that already discussed for electronic focussing. If the transmitter drive pulse to each element is delayed by an increasing amount with increasing distance across the array, then the transmitted pulse is emitted first from the element with the shortest delay and last from the element with the longest delay at the other end of the array. The wavefronts are then inclined to the transducer face as shown and the beam is emitted at an angle to the perpendicular to the transducer face. Changing the range of delay across the array will alter the beam orientation. Thus the beam can be swept through a sector-shaped scan.

7.5.2 Focussing

Focussing can be achieved by incorporating a degree of curvature in the increase of delay with array element number as shown in Figure 7.16b. As with the linear array scanner the electronic focussing takes place only within the scan plane. Slice width reduction requires shaping of the elements or the use of a cylindrical lens. Similar delays can be used to beam-steer and focus during reception, and multiple zone focussing, dynamic focussing, apodisation and aperture control can all be used as with the annular and linear arrays.

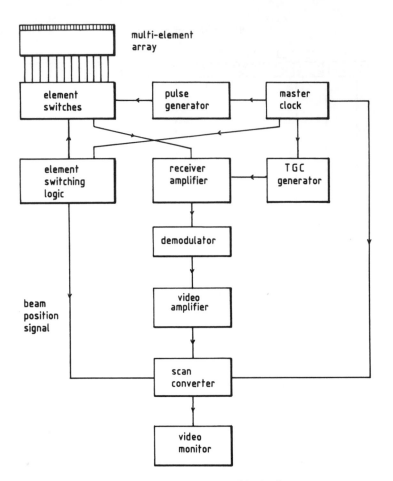

Figure 7.12 Linear array scanner block diagram.

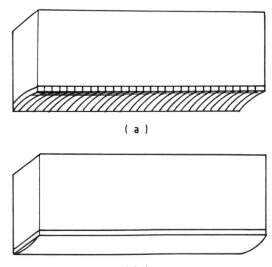

Figure 7.13 Focussing to achieve slice width reduction using shaped transducer elements (a) and cylindrical lens (b).

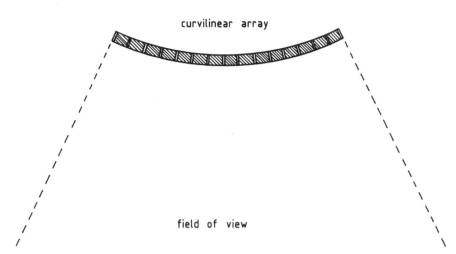

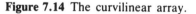

Figure 7.14 The curvilinear array.

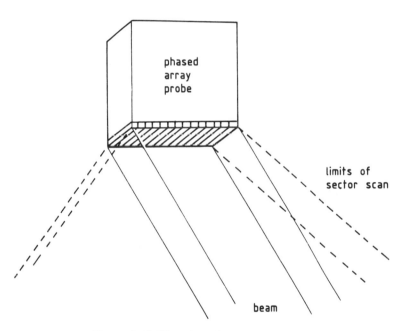

Figure 7.15 The phased array probe.

7.5.3 Block Diagram

Clearly the delay mechanisms may be similar to those for these other transducer types; only the delay control logic has a different architecture. The phased array scanner therefore has the same parts as a static B-scanner with the delays and delay control that we have seen in use in the annular array incorporated (Figure 7.17). The beam orientation signal required by the scan converter in this case comes from the delay controller.

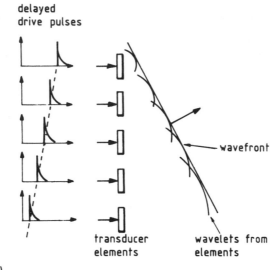

(a)

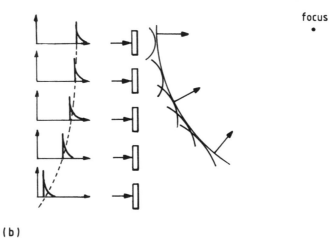

(b)

Figure 7.16 Electronic beam steering (a) and beam steering combined with focussing (b). Note that the drive pulses are shown plotted against time whereas the wavefronts are shown as a 'snapshot' view.

7.5.4 Aperture Reduction

Unlike the other scanners, the beam from a phased array scanner is not always perpendicular to the transducer face. This means that the effective aperture of the transducer decreases as the beam direction angle increases, resulting in a decrease in the near zone and increase in far zone beam divergence (Figure 7.18).

7.6 GRATING LOBES

In addition to side lobes (reduced by apodisation) the phased and linear array scanners also generate

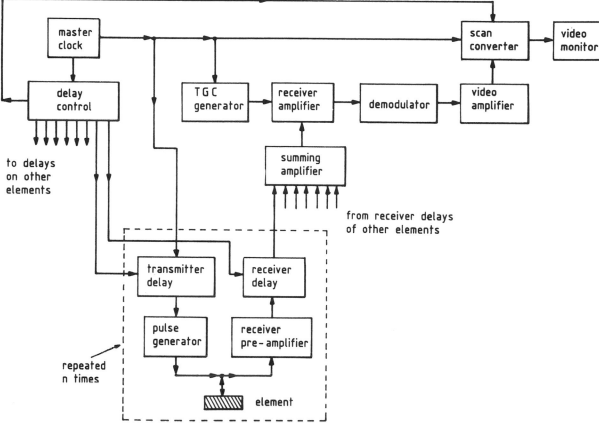

Figure 7.17 Phased array scanner block diagram.

lobes in the beam as a result of interference of the ultrasound from the regularly spaced elements. The lobes are called grating lobes and are qualitatively similar to the side lobes already discussed. They may be reduced by increasing the number of elements while keeping the length of the array the same (i.e. reducing the element size).

7.7 PROBE CONSTRUCTION

There are some considerations which are similar for all the real-time scanners. The probes all have some parts in common with the A-scan probe. They all need absorbing, high-attenuation backing, electrical screening, acoustic insulation from

the case, matching layers and electrical connections. The multi-element transducers may have acoustic insulation between elements to avoid the vibration of one being passed on to neighbours.

7.8 FRAME RATE

The constraints on pulse repetition frequency are the same as for the A-scan instrument, but in the case of the real-time scanner, the beam moves to the next position in the scan sequence before the next transmitter pulse. Thus the scan rate is related to the PRF by:

Scan (Frame) rate

$$= \text{PRF}/(\text{Number of scan lines}) \quad (7.1)$$

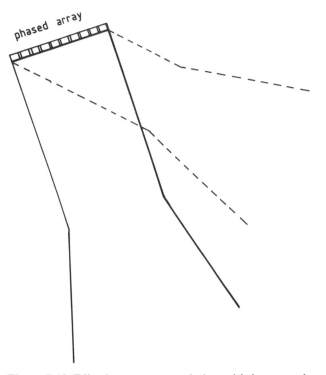

Figure 7.18 Effective aperture variation with beam angle.

The frame rate should be at least 20 per second in order to avoid image flicker. Since the PRF is limited by the maximum depth (equation 5.3) there is a limit to the number of scan lines. Consideration must be given to the spacing of these lines. Increasing the spacing will increase the width of the scan for a given number of scan lines, but if the line separation is comparable with the beam width, then lateral resolution will be degraded. A design example is considered in Appendix I.

7.9 INSTRUMENT COMPARISON

In conclusion, it is worth comparing the different types of instrument.

The mechanical scanner is electronically simple, has a complex moving mechanism, has a circular transducer allowing focussing perpendicular to the scan plane (slice thickness reduction) in addition to focussing in the scan plane, vibrates and requires a large probe. The mechanical sector scanner requires a small acoustic window but has a small width of scan close to the probe.

The linear array scanner has an equal width scan at all depths but a large acoustic window is required, an even larger transducer, more complex electronics, no moving parts and the facility for simultaneous M-mode (see Chapter 8). The curvilinear array scan is a compromise between the advantages and disadvantages of sector and rectilinear scans.

The phased array scanner requires much more complex electronics (expense), no moving parts, has a sector scan (small acoustic window required) and has a smaller, lighter probe than the mechanical sector scanner. The aperture varies with the angle of beam deviation and therefore the resolution tends to be poorer than for the mechanical sector scanner. The instrument can also incorporate a simultaneous M-mode facility.

CHAPTER 8

M-Mode

8.1 INTRODUCTION

M-mode, also known as TM (Time Motion) and TP (Time Position) scanning, is a means of indicating tissue movement with time. It is most often used for cardiac measurements, particularly for detecting abnormalities in the movement of heart valves.

8.2 CONSTRUCTION AND OPERATION

The simplest M-mode scanner is shown in Figure 8.1, from which it can be seen that most of the instrument is similar to a normal A-scan instrument. The principle of operation is indicated in Figure 8.2. A brightness-modulated display, similar to a single B-scan line, is written vertically on the screen and this display line is moved slowly across the screen at a regular rate, so that stationary reflectors are indicated by horizontal lines whilst the variation in position with time of moving reflectors is indicated by the vertical movement of their echo on the screen.

8.3 DISPLAY AND RECORDING MODES

8.3.1 Scroll and Sweep Displays

The type of display shown here is limited since the display from only a few cardiac cycles can be shown before the trace reaches the side of the screen and the process has to be repeated. If a scan converter and video display are used, then

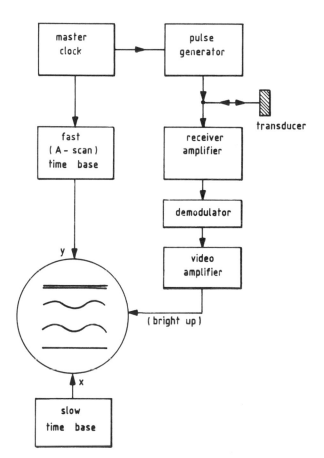

Figure 8.1 M-mode scanner block diagram.

either the display can be as shown above (sweep mode) or the previously acquired information can be displayed by moving the whole waveform across the screen and adding information from the most recent A-scan on one side of the screen.

97

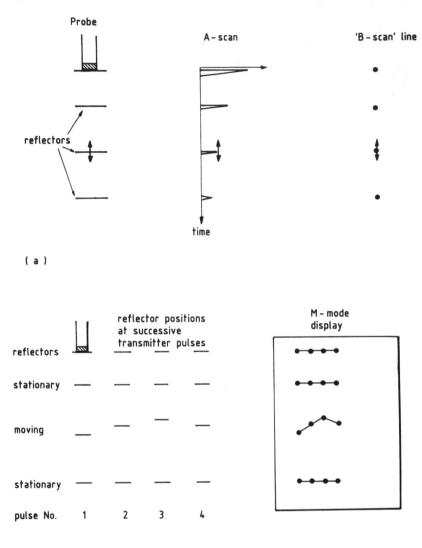

Figure 8.2 M-mode display generation. Probe/reflector geometry, A-scan and B-scan line (a) and successive-pulse reflector positions and display (b).

This is termed the scroll mode. The two methods are shown in Figure 8.3. In the scroll mode, it is possible to change the transducer orientation while imaging and simply freeze the display when the required waveforms are obtained. It is also possible to store several seconds of information and replay the traces later. Data recording in these cases can be by photographic record of one or more screen-fulls of information or a video recording of information obtained in the scroll mode.

8.3.2 UV Recording

A method of recording allowing the viewing of relatively long records is shown in Figure 8.4. In this case, the single intensity-modulated line

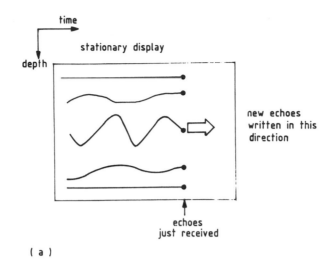

(a)

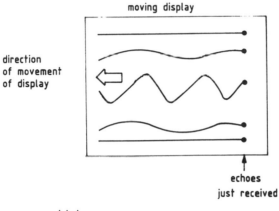

(b)

Figure 8.3 Display during sweep mode (a) and scroll mode (b).

remains constant on the screen and this display is transferred by optical fibres to a moving light-sensitive paper. The latent image generated is fully developed by irradiation using an ultraviolet (UV) lamp.

8.3.3 Sweep Speed

In all these methods, the time base or chart speed can be altered to allow a large number of cycles of information per screen (or per unit length of chart recorder paper) or a faster time base or chart recorder speed can be used to allow the examination of individual cycles in detail.

8.3.4 Measurement

Time, distances of movement and speed of movement of reflectors can be measured from the trace as indicated in Figure 8.5.

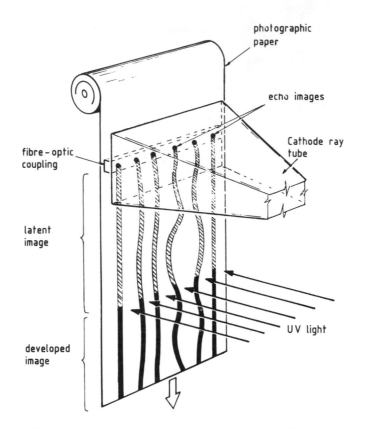

Figure 8.4 Formation of the M-mode display using a UV recorder.

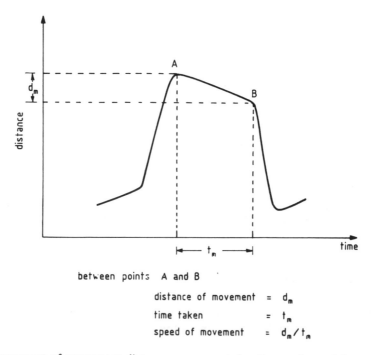

between points A and B

distance of movement = d_m
time taken = t_m
speed of movement = d_m / t_m

Figure 8.5 Measurement of movement distance, movement duration and speed from an M-mode trace.

8.4 COMBINATION M- AND B-MODE

M-mode displays can be used on static B-scanners by simply switching to this display mode when the beam is passing through the area of interest as indicated on the B-scan image. A real-time display can be frozen, the beam steered to the appropriate place on the image and the M-mode displayed—often on the same display by sharing the scan converter. Simultaneous B-mode and M-mode displays can be generated, with phased array scanners, by switching to the M-mode beam every few image lines. The image build-up is indicated in Figure 8.6. There is obviously a reduction in frame rate or sector size associated with this, depending on the rate of update of the M-mode display. This rapid change of beam direction cannot be achieved using a mechanical sector scanner because of mechanical inertia.

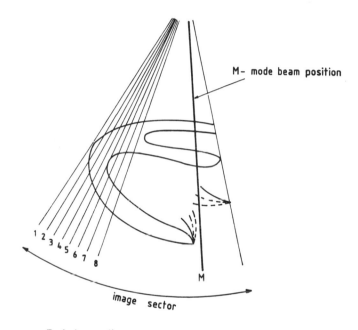

Typical scan line sequence
12M34M56M78 etc.

Figure 8.6 Scan line sequence during simultaneous sector and M-mode display.

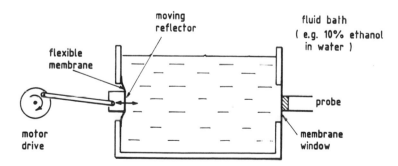

Figure 8.7 M-mode calibration rig.

8.5 PULSE REPETITION FREQUENCY

A reasonably high pulse repetition frequency is required in order to follow adequately high-velocity reflectors. For example, sampling reflectors moving at 300 mm/s and allowing half a millimetre of travel between samples requires a PRF of 600 Hz. Accuracies of distance of travel movement of $\pm$ 0.5 mm and time measurement to 10 ms or better are required for cardiac scanning.

8.6 TEST OBJECT

A suitable test object for M-mode scanners is a motor-driven reflector, for example that shown in Figure 8.7. If this has a known variation of position with time, then the accuracy of the display can be assessed.

CHAPTER 9

Other Scanners and Probes

9.1 INTRODUCTION

In this brief chapter we consider those scanners and probes which do not fit neatly into the categories discussed elsewhere.

9.2 C-MODE

The C-mode or constant depth scanner samples the echo return a fixed time after each transmitted pulse. It therefore generates a signal indicating the reflections or scatter from a particular depth in tissue. A water bath technique is used and the transducer is moved in a raster (or spiral fashion) as shown in Figure 9.1 and the echo return is indicated as a brightness-modulated display against transducer position. The display is therefore similar to a B-scan display except that the image plane is perpendicular to the beam. This type of scanner has seen little clinical use.

9.3 PLAN POSITION INDICATION (PPI) SCANNING

PPI scanning is used in intracavity probes. The beam is moved repetitively round in a circle about the axis of the probe and echo intensity is shown plotted against depth (radial position) and angle of rotation (Figure 9.2). The beam can be generated from a side-facing transducer mounted on a motor-driven rod rotating within an oil-filled outer sheath. Alternatively, a circumferential array of transducer elements can be used to sweep the beam by switching elements in a similar fashion to that used in a linear array (Figure 9.2b).

9.4 OTHER INTRACAVITY PROBES

End-view and side-view sector scans can be performed using small phased arrays and side-view rectilinear scans using small linear arrays on intracavity probes (Figure 9.3). Sector scans may be performed using small rocking transducers.

The advantage of using the intracavity probes is that organs close to the cavity can be imaged using a higher frequency, and therefore better resolution can be obtained than when using standard abdominal scanning. In addition, shadowing, due to bowel gas, can be avoided.

9.5 INTRAOPERATIVE PROBES

Small high-frequency (8–15 MHz) sector and linear array probes can be used for imaging organs by direct contact. To avoid dead zone problems, it may be necessary to use a standoff arrangement. The probes themselves may be fluid sterilised and covered by a sterile thin plastic or latex sheath.

9.6 BIOPSY PROBES

Biopsy needles can be positioned under ultrasound guidance using a probe with a needle

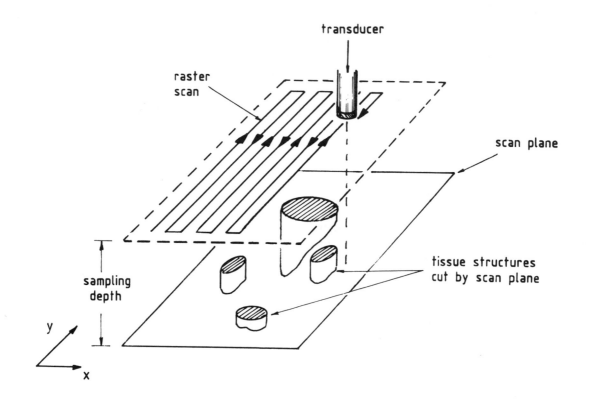

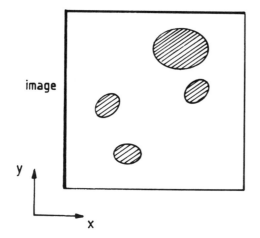

Figure 9.1 C-scan probe movement and image.

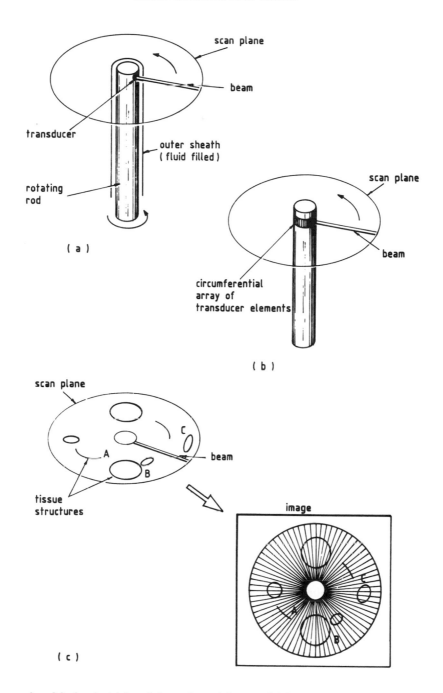

Figure 9.2 PPI scanning. Mechanical (a) and circumferential array. (b) Beam/reflector geometry and corresponding image (c).

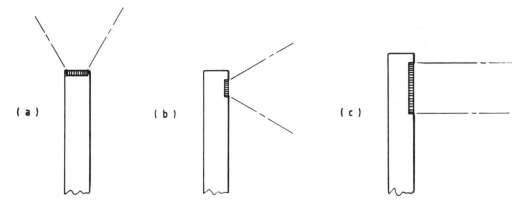

Figure 9.3 Array transducer arrangements in intracavity probes. End-view phased array (a), side-view phased array (b) and side-view linear array (c).

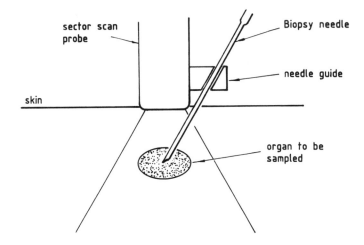

Figure 9.4 Biopsy attachment to a sector scan probe.

guide. A real-time mechanical sector scanner with a needle guide is shown in Figure 9.4. Similar guides can be used with linear array probes. The needle tip is a strong scatterer of ultrasound and is clearly visible on the ultrasound image, enabling accurate positioning within the organ to be sampled.

CHAPTER 10

Measurement of Size

10.1 INTRODUCTION

Measurement of size is used to determine whether or not a tissue structure is within the normal size range. It is used, for example, to detect an abnormal fetal growth pattern and abnormal cardiac chamber size. It is used, together with blood velocity measurement, to calculate blood flow rate in order to determine whether organ perfusion is adequate.

10.2 MEASUREMENT FROM THE A-SCAN

The distance between interfaces can be measured on an A-scan by noting the distance between the echoes on the horizontal axis of the display. A more convenient method is by using electronically generated caliper markers which are usually bright spots set to the leading edges of the echoes concerned (Figure 10.1). A suitable block diagram is shown in Figure 10.2. The master timer and

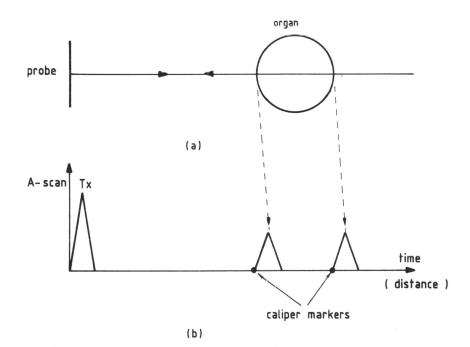

Figure 10.1 Electronic caliper measurements on an A-scan display. Probe/organ geometry (a) and caliper marker positioning (b).

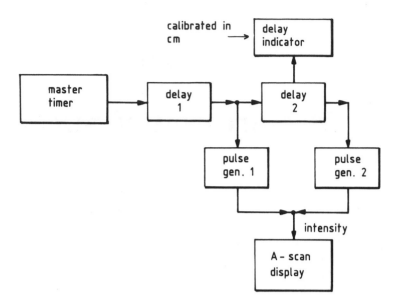

Figure 10.2 A-scan electronic caliper block diagram.

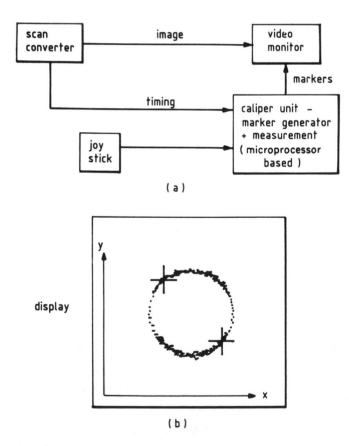

Figure 10.3 B-scan electronic caliper. Block diagram (a) and linear measurement display (b).

A-scan display are those of the existing A-scan instrument and the rest of the unit is the caliper. After a delay (1) following the transmitter pulse, the pulse generator (1) is triggered and intensifies a spot on the A-scan display. Delay (1) is altered by an operator to place the bright spot on the leading edge of the first echo. Following a further delay (2) the pulse generator (2) is triggered and this again intensifies the A-scan display, giving rise to a bright spot on the screen, the position of which is adjusted by altering delay (2) until it is coincident with the leading edge of the second echo. Delay (2) is then proportional to the distance between the two interfaces and the delay can be indicated on a separate display calibrated in distance. Thus every 13 μs of delay will be indicated as 1 cm on the display.

10.3 MEASUREMENT FROM THE B-SCAN

10.3.1 Measurement from Hard Copy

Measurements can be made from a hard copy using a ruler for linear measurement, a planimeter for area measurement and a map wheel for circumference. These methods are time-consuming and also susceptible to geometrical distortion on the display.

10.3.2 Electronic Measurement

An electronic caliper can be quickly used and any distortion in the display will affect both the calipers and the image equally and therefore give rise to no error in measurement. The block diagram of the caliper unit plus a display is shown in Figure 10.3. The scan converter and video monitor are those of the B-scanner. The joystick and caliper unit are used for measurement. The caliper unit is usually based on a microprocessor. Timing information from the scan converter will tell the caliper unit the position of the spot on the video monitor. The joystick will allow the operator to position markers (usually crosses) generated by the caliper unit and displayed on the video monitor.

10.3.3 Linear Measurement

For simple linear measurement the operator will place one caliper marker at one end of the distance to be measured. The unit is then told to store this position (by pressing a key, e.g. 'ENTER'). The first marker will then be stored in position and the x and y co-ordinates of the marker will be stored in the microprocessor unit. The second caliper will then be positioned at the end of the distance to be measured, and the unit will calculate the co-ordinates of this position and the distance between the two caliper markers, and display the result.

10.3.4 Non-Linear Measurement

Non-linear measurements can be carried out as illustrated in Figure 10.4. One marker is placed at the beginning of the structure to be measured and the second marker moved along the structure while the caliper unit marks its progress by secondary markers, usually bright spots, at regular intervals. The total distance is then calculated by the unit as the sum of the distances between the secondary markers. This can be extended to circumference measurement as illustrated in Figure 10.5, where the second marker is moved completely round the perimeter of the object until it coincides with the first.

10.3.5 Area Measurement

A method of area measurement is illustrated in Figure 10.6. The second marker is moved round the perimeter of the area to be measured and the unit calculates the areas of rectangles of heights equal to the y-co-ordinate at each secondary marker and of width equal to the horizontal spacings of the markers. The areas of these rectangles are added together for increasing x and subtracted from the total for decreasing x. The net area is that of the multiple straight line approximation to the true area shown in Figure 10.7. The method has been illustrated using a

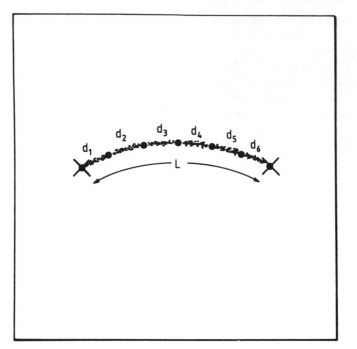

$$L = d_1 + d_2 + d_3 + d_4 + d_5 + d_6$$

Figure 10.4 Non-linear measurement display and calculation.

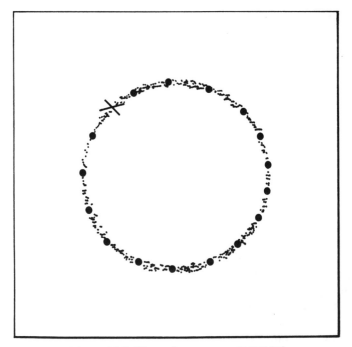

Figure 10.5 Circumference measurement.

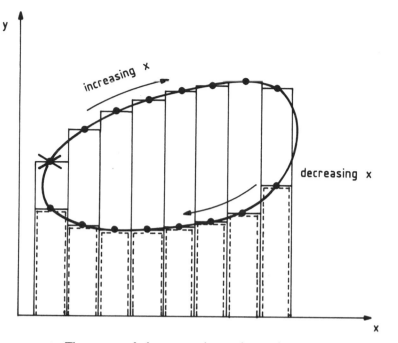

Figure 10.6 Area measurement. The areas of the rectangles under each measurement point are added for increasing x and subtracted for decreasing x.

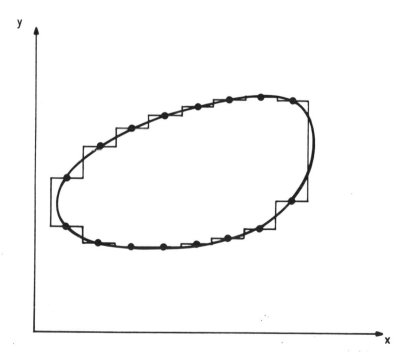

Figure 10.7 Approximation to organ perimeter used in area measurement.

cartesian co-ordinate system but the method works equally well using polar co-ordinates.

Areas may also be calculated from linear measurements by assuming an area shape. For example, if a circular shape may be assumed, the area may be calculated from a diameter (D) measurement:

$$\text{Area} = \frac{\pi D^2}{4} \qquad (10.1)$$

If an ellipse is assumed, the area may be calculated from the largest (D_1) and smallest (D_2) dimension measurement:

$$\text{Area} = \frac{\pi D_1 D_2}{4} \qquad (10.2)$$

10.3.6 Volume Measurement

Three methods of volume measurement are shown in Figure 10.8. The first two methods approximate the volume of the organ to a particular geometric shape—an ellipsoid in Figure 10.8a and half an ellipsoid in Figure 10.8b. In both cases the volume is:

$$V = \frac{\pi}{6} D_1 D_2^2 \qquad (10.3)$$

The third method (Figure 10.8c) involves taking a number of parallel sectional images of the organ to be measured, measuring the cross-sectional areas and adding the volumes of the cylinders of cross-sectional area equal to the areas measured and height equal to the scan separation.

If the cross-sectional areas are $A_1, A_2 \ldots A_n$ then the volume is:

$$V = h (A_1 + A_2 \ldots A_n) \qquad (10.4)$$

If the areas are calculated from diameters assuming circular cross-sections then:

$$V = \frac{\pi h}{4} (D_1^2 + D_2^2 \ldots D_h^2) \qquad (10.5)$$

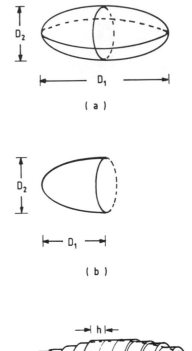

(a)

(b)

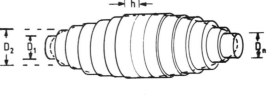

(c)

Figure 10.8 Volume measurement. Approximation to an elipsoid (a) and a semi-elipsoid (b). Multiple cylinder approximation method using cross-sectional area measurements from parallel cross-sectional images (c).

10.4 ERRORS IN MEASUREMENT

10.4.1 Calibration Velocity

Obviously, depth measurement will be in error if the velocity in the tissue between two points is different from the calibration velocity of the caliper unit. The measured distance will be smaller if the characteristic velocity is higher than the calibration velocity and *vice versa*. The error is illustrated in Figure 10.9. Obviously, only depth

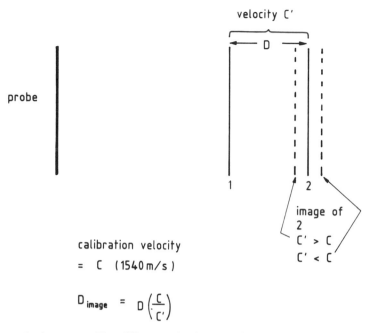

Figure 10.9 Calibration velocity error. The difference in the velocity of the ultrasound between two interfaces and the caliper calibration velocity will give rise to a distance measurement error.

measurement is affected in this way by velocity changes since distances measured perpendicular to the beams across the scan plane in a linear array scan are defined by the geometry of the probe. This is illustrated in Figure 10.10. For a sector scan (Figure 10.11) the depth measurement is made along radial beam positions and these measurements will be affected by velocity. In this case angular displacements about the axis of rotation of the transducer will be unaffected by velocity changes. Normally measurements will not be made exactly along the ultrasound beam direction and measurements at an angle to this direction will be partially affected by velocity changes.

10.4.2 Refraction

Velocity differences will also cause errors via the phenomenon of refraction. This is illustrated in Figure 10.12.

10.4.3 Cursor Placement

A major source of error in measuring small distances is error in placement of the cursors. This is related to the resolution of the image and will be affected by beam width, axial resolution, image pixel size and displayed echo amplitude. Measurement of the internal diameter of blood vessels for reasons of blood flow measurement can be in error due to the multi-layer nature of the blood vessel wall. The blood-vessel wall boundary may be easily identified on the distal wall but the proximal wall image will be complicated by overlapping echoes from the multiple layers, leading to an uncertainty as to the position of the blood–wall interface. This is particularly important when the cross-sectional area of the vessel is calculated from the diameter measurement. Since this involves a squaring of the diameter, any error in the diameter measurement will be doubled as a percentage error in the area.

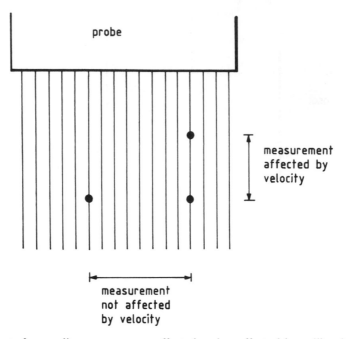

measurement
affected by
velocity

measurement
not affected
by velocity

Figure 10.10 Measurements from a linear array scan affected and unaffected by calibration velocity errors.

10.4.4 Caliper Resolution

Frequently distances are displayed only to two-figure accuracy and this can have a significant effect on the accuracy of the measurement. There are two methods of determining the least significant displayed digit; the first one is truncation. In this case any numbers less significant than the first two are simply dropped when the number is displayed (e.g. 8.57 is displayed as 8.5). In this case the percentage error can be up to 10% (10.99 displayed as 10). The other method of last-digit calculation is called round-off and in this case the least significant digit is displayed as

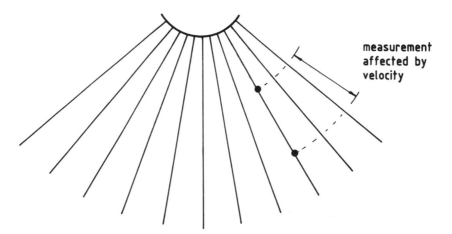

measurement
affected by
velocity

Figure 10.11 Calibration velocity error—distance affected in a sector scan.

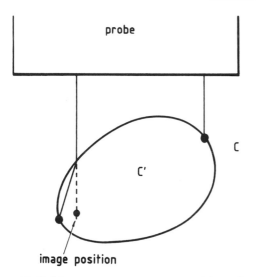

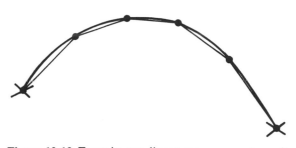

Figure 10.13 Error in non-linear measurement resulting from piecewise linear approximation.

Figure 10.12 Measurement error resulting from refraction.

the nearest number to the calculated number (e.g. 8.57 displayed as 8.6) and the percentage error ranges up to 5% (10.499 displayed as 10).

10.4.5 Caliper Accuracy

It is possible for the caliper calibration of the instrument to be in error. It is worth checking the caliper accuracy periodically using wire reflectors in a medium of normal characteristic velocity.

10.4.6 Patient Movement

Obviously if there is patient movement between the start and the end of a measurement there will be an error. This is not a problem when measuring from a frozen image.

10.4.7 Non-Linear and Circumference Measurement

The number of sample points along a curve will give rise to an error if this number is small. This is illustrated in Figure 10.13. The sum of the

distances along the piecewise straight line approximation is obviously less than the distance along the curve and this error will be larger if the number of points is reduced. The instrument may well use an algorithm which takes into account curvature by drawing curves through three points at a time rather than straight lines joining two as shown. This will reduce the error but not remove it altogether. There will also be an operator-induced error in tracing a curve or perimeter as shown in Figure 10.14. This will, in general, give rise to a higher measured perimeter.

10.4.8 Area Measurement

Area measurements will be affected by the same measurement errors as linear and non-linear

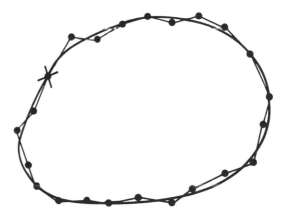

Figure 10.14 Operator error in tracing organ perimeter.

measurements. In general, the tracing errors will tend to cancel and therefore not be as great as for perimeter measurement.

Calculations of area from linear distance measurement assuming a particular shape (e.g. circle or ellipse) will be in error if the actual shape is different from that assumed.

As mentioned in Section 10.4.3, errors in area calculation from a single diameter of a circle will have approximately twice the percentage error as that of the diameter measurement.

10.4.9 Volume Measurement

Volume measurements are made using linear and area measurements and therefore suffer from the same errors as these separate measurements. The other errors are related to the algorithm used. Referring to Figure 10.8 in the multiple cylinder method, there are no assumptions as to the shape of the volume involved but the degree to which the model is a good approximation to the volume to be measured will increase with the number of cylinders. Unfortunately, the error due to the sum of the errors in all the area measurements will increase if the number of cylinders increases. The accuracy will also depend on the slice separation being maintained accurately throughout the whole volume. The method is obviously particularly sensitive to patient movement. The other two methods depend on an approximation of a standard geometrical shape to the volume being measured and there will be some error according to the degree of approximation.

CHAPTER 11

Doppler Ultrasound Physics and Instruments

11.1 DOPPLER EFFECT

The Doppler effect is a shift in the observed frequency of a radiated wave motion when there is relative movement between the source of the radiation and the observer. A now classic example is that of the police car siren which sounds higher pitched when a car is travelling towards you than when the car is stationary and lower pitched when the car is travelling away.

11.1.1 Moving Source

With reference to Figure 11.1a, if both the source and the observer are stationary then the crests of the waves, which are emitted at a regular rate (the transmission frequency), travel through the intervening medium at constant speed, each crest spaced from its neighbour by the wavelength, and pass the observer at the same rate transmitted. If, however, the source is moving towards the stationary observer (Figure 11.1b) the source moves a short distance towards the observer between the emission of each crest. This means that the crests are spaced closer together. In effect the wavelength has shortened. These crests pass the observer at the same speed but since they are closer together, the observer experiences a higher frequency. Conversely, if the source is moving away from the observer the wavelength is increased and the observer will experience a lower frequency.

11.1.2 Moving Observer

If the source is stationary and the observer is moving towards the source (Figure 11.1c) then the observer will intercept the crests at a faster rate. The observer will thus experience a higher frequency. Conversely, if the observer is moving away from the source then the observer will intercept the crests at a lower rate and will experience a lower frequency. In the case of both the moving source and the moving observer, the difference between the received and transmitted frequencies is known as the Doppler shift.

11.1.3 Moving Reflector

In medical Doppler ultrasound instruments both the source (the transmitting transducer) and the observer (receiving transducer) are mounted in a probe and are stationary with respect to the medium (tissue). Any reflector or scatterer of ultrasound can be considered as first an observer of the transmitted ultrasound and then as a source of ultrasound for the receiver. If the scatterer or reflector is stationary then the receiver picks up scattered ultrasound at the same frequency as that transmitted (Figure 11.2a). However, if the scatterer is moving away from the ultrasound probe (Figure 11.2b) then, first as an observer of the transmitted ultrasound it will see a lower frequency than that transmitted, and then as a source for the receiving transducer it will emit

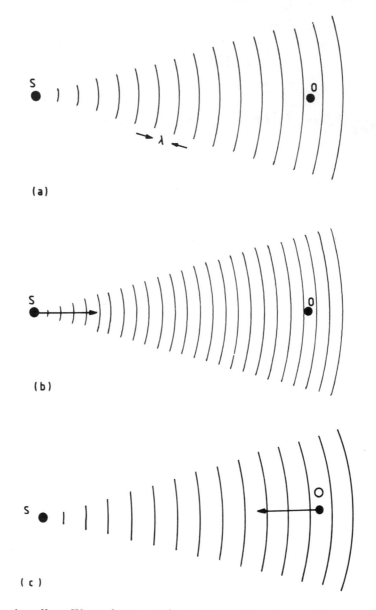

Figure 11.1 The Doppler effect. Waves from a stationary source S passing a stationary observer O (a). Source moving towards the observer (b) and observer moving towards source (c).

ultrasound of a longer wavelength than it has observed. Thus in the case of the moving reflector or scatterer, there are two Doppler shifts in the same direction and the observer will experience a lower frequency than that transmitted. Conversely, if the scatterer is moving towards the probe the observer will experience a higher frequency than that transmitted. The Doppler shift (the difference between the observed and the transmitted frequency) is proportional to the velocity of the scatterer. In medical Doppler ultrasound the scatterer (e.g. a red blood cell) is often moving at an angle to the transmitter and receiver beams and this situation is illustrated in

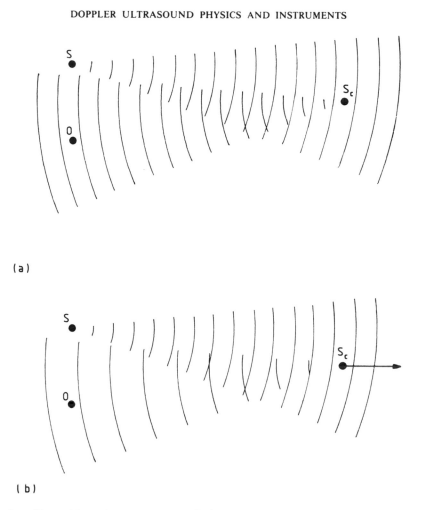

(a)

(b)

Figure 11.2 Doppler effect with stationary source and observer and moving scatterer S_c. Stationary scatterer (a) and scatterer moving away from source and observer (b).

Figure 11.3. The Doppler shift frequency is given by:

$$f_d = \frac{-2Vf_0 \cos(\theta) \cos(\delta/2)}{c} \quad (11.1)$$

where

V = scatterer velocity
f_0 = transmitted frequency
c = speed of ultrasound
θ = angle between the bisector of the transmitter and receiver beams and the direction of movement
δ = angle between the transmitter and receiver beams

The negative sign indicates that the Doppler shift is negative (transmitted frequency shifted to a lower frequency) if the direction of movement is in the conventionally positive direction (away from the transducers).

The angle (δ) between the beams is usually sufficiently small that $\cos(\delta/2)$ is close to 1.0. In pulsed Doppler instruments (described later) the same transducer is used for transmission and reception and $\delta = 0$ ($\cos(\delta/2) = 1$). Thus the above equation may be simplified to:

$$f_d = \frac{-2Vf_0 \cos(\theta)}{c} \quad (11.2)$$

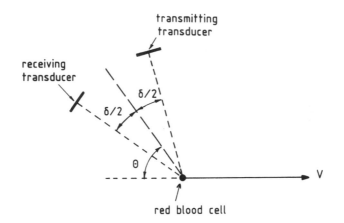

Figure 11.3 Continuous wave (CW) Doppler ultrasound transducer arrangement. Reproduced by permission, from Fish, P.J. (1981) Recent advances in cardio-vascular Doppler. In: A Kurjak (ed.) *Progress in Medical Ultrasound*, Vol. 2, Elsevier.

Note that there is no Doppler shift ($f_d = 0$) if $\theta = 90°$ (cos $\theta = 0$) and the Doppler shift increases as θ decreases from 90° to 0°.

The transmitted frequency is usually in the range 2–10 MHz depending on the required penetration. In the Doppler instruments used to detect blood flow the determination of this frequency is from consideration of the trade-off between increasing attenuation and increasing backscatter from the blood cells (scattered intensity proportional to f_0^4 as the frequency increases.

The velocities of interest are usually such that the Doppler shift frequencies are in the audible range (100 Hz to 15 kHz) and it is usual to provide some means of listening to the Doppler shift signals.

11.2 DOPPLER FREQUENCY EXTRACTION—THE DOPPLER DEMODULATOR

Since we are interested in the shift in frequency (this shift being proportional to velocity) it is convenient to generate a signal having this frequency. Methods of achieving this are illustrated in Figures 11.4 and 11.5. In the first method (Figure 11.4) the transmitted and received signals are added together, and, because the signals are of different frequency, they move in and out of phase, constructive interference resulting in a maxima of the signals when they are in phase and destructive interference resulting in a minima when the signals are out of phase. The envelope of the resulting signal has a 'beat frequency' equal to the difference between the frequencies. Demodulating this signal (rectifying and passing through a filter (a low-pass filter—see Appendix E) to remove the high-frequency components) will result in a signal (the Doppler signal) having a frequency equal to the Doppler shift. In the alternative method (Figure 11.5) the transmitted and received signals are multiplied, and filtered to remove the high-frequency components in order to derive the Doppler signal.

11.3 THE CONTINUOUS WAVE DOPPLER INSTRUMENT

11.3.1 Construction and Operation

The continuous wave Doppler instrument is shown in its most common form as a blood flow detector in Figure 11.6. The transmitting transducer (T) is connected to an oscillator and transmits ultrasound continuously. The ultrasound reflected and scattered from tissue structures is picked up by the receiving transducer (R) mounted in the same probe. The electrical output

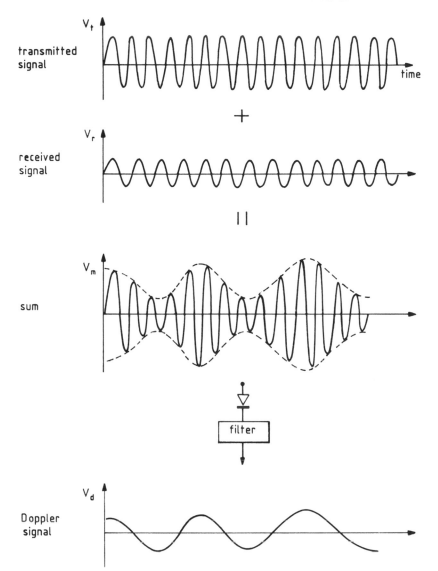

Figure 11.4 Doppler demodulation by summation, rectification and filtering.

from this transducer is amplified and fed to the Doppler demodulator where it is mixed with a signal (the reference signal) from the transmitter oscillator, and the resulting Doppler signal is amplified and fed to loudspeakers or headphones and a frequency meter.

Since there is a range of blood velocities in any one blood vessel, the Doppler signal contains a range of frequencies corresponding to a range of blood velocities and as a result sounds noise-like.

The velocity of blood within vessels also varies with time. The blood velocity in arteries has a regular pulsation corresponding to the heartbeat and the velocity in veins often varies with respiration. Typical tracings obtained from a chart recorder coupled to the output of the frequency meter are shown in Figure 11.7.

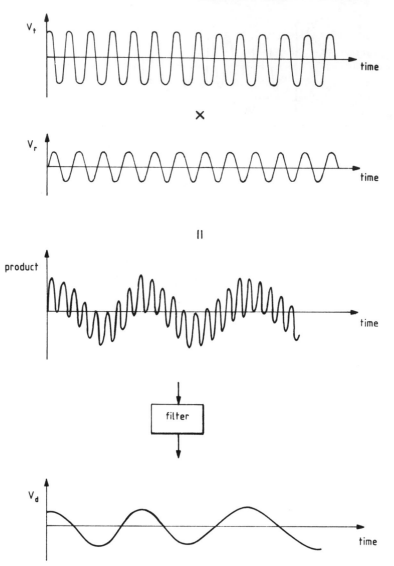

Figure 11.5 Doppler demodulation by multiplication and filtering.

Other structures in the body may move with breathing or heartbeat and these movements will give rise to high-amplitude but usually low-frequency Doppler shift signals. In particular, when looking at arteries, the signal from the vessel walls will give rise to high-amplitude, low-frequency Doppler signals (Figure 11.8) and these will tend to overload amplifiers used to boost the small signal from the red blood cells. The Doppler signal from the Doppler demodulator therefore is high-pass filtered to remove these low-frequency signals (below about 200 Hz) before amplification. This filter is often known as the 'wall thump filter'. The Doppler signal also passes through a low-pass filter which limits the frequencies passed to the frequency meter to just above

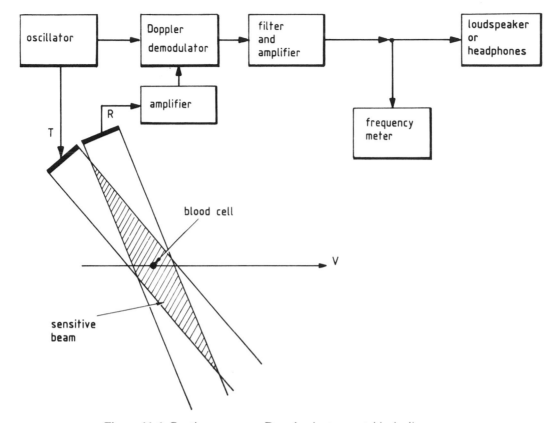

Figure 11.6 Continuous wave Doppler instrument block diagram.

the maximum expected Doppler frequency. This limits the background noise to this maximum frequency, so reducing the power of the interfering noise.

Because ultrasound is being transmitted continuously and the same transducer cannot be used for reception there are two transducers and the instrument is sensitive to blood flow within the region of overlap of the two beams. The angle between the receiver and transmitter beams is usually fairly small, resulting in a useful length of sensitive beam.

The sensitive beam of instruments used for peripheral vessel monitoring is usually a few millimetres wide in order to allow for the monitoring of signals from single vessels. It will be somewhat larger in instruments designed for use on the thoracic aorta, for example.

The construction of the probe of a continuous wave Doppler instrument for blood flow detection is shown in Figure 11.9. Note that no backing is required since the transducer is not pulsed.

A sensitive beam width of a few centimetres is required in instruments used for fetal heart detection and monitoring in order to enable quick location of the fetal heart and allow for fetal movement without the heart moving outside the sensitive beam. This wide sensitive beam is often achieved by the use of a number of transducers with overlapping beams, within the Doppler probe.

11.3.2 Flow Direction Discrimination

The instrument described so far will not discriminate between flow directions. Although flow

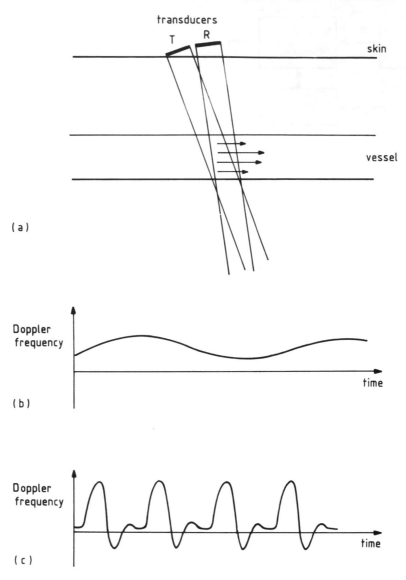

Figure 11.7 Transducer/vessel geometry (a), Doppler frequency waveform from a vein (b) and an artery (c).

away from the probe will give rise to a negative Doppler shift (received frequency lower than transmitted frequency) and flow towards the probe will give rise to a positive Doppler shift (received frequency higher than transmitted frequency) the Doppler signal delivered by a simple instrument will be the same in both cases. There are two main methods of achieving a directional instrument (Figure 11.10).

In the first (Figure 11.10a) the Doppler demodulator is given a reference signal with a frequency equal to the oscillator frequency minus an offset. In this case all the Doppler signals are shifted in frequency by this offset; positive Doppler shifts appearing above the offset frequency and negative Doppler shifts below the offset frequency.

The second method (Figure 11.10b) involves

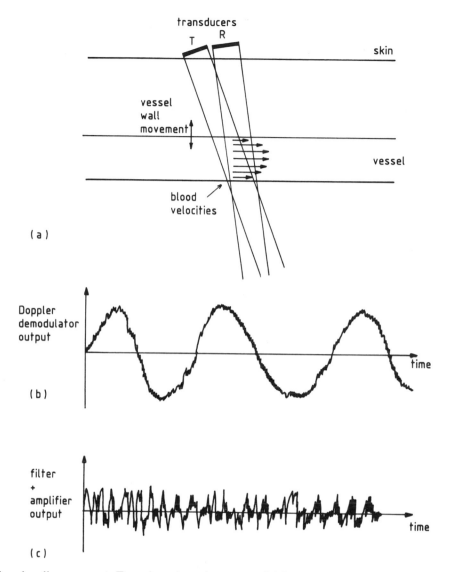

Figure 11.8 Vessel wall movement. Transducer/vessel geometry (a) Doppler demodulator (mixer) output (b) and high-pass filtered and amplified demodulator output (c).

two Doppler demodulators together with their associated filters and amplifiers. The reference to one is from the oscillator as before. This is known as the in-phase reference. The second has a reference which is 90° phase shifted and this reference is known as the quadrature reference. The Doppler signals at the outputs of the two Doppler signal amplifiers are therefore 90° phase shifted with respect to each other but the phase shift will be in one direction for positive Doppler shifts and in the other direction for negative Doppler shifts. The direction of flow can therefore be detected by a phase detector coupled to the outputs of these two amplifiers. The output of the phase detector can be used to alter the polarity of the output of the frequency meter in order to correctly indicate positive or negative velocities.

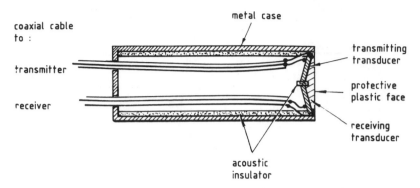

Figure 11.9 Continuous wave Doppler instrument probe.

11.4 THE PULSED DOPPLER INSTRUMENT

11.4.1 Introduction

The major limitation of the continuous wave instrument is that it is sensitive to flow in the whole region of overlap of the two ultrasound beams, although in practice it is usually limited in depth by attenuation. This means that there is no separation of signals from two or more vessels in the beam and there is no separation of signals from different parts of the same vessel. To overcome this problem, we need an instrument with range resolution and this is provided by the pulsed Doppler flow detector.

11.4.2 Construction and Operation

A block diagram of the instrument is shown in Figure 11.11. As with the pulsed imaging instruments, a single transducer may be used for both transmission and reception. The transducer is driven during transmission by a short burst of signal from the oscillator when the timing circuits open the gate between the oscillator and the transducer. Ultrasound is backscattered to the receiving transducer, as before, amplified and passed to the Doppler demodulator but in this case the output of the demodulator is not monitored continuously but sampled by opening a gate after a delay following the transmitter pulse. The transmission and demodulator sampling takes place periodically at the pulse repetition frequency. The process for a single reflector is illustrated in Figure 11.12.

As the reflector moves away from the transducer as shown in Figure 11.12a, the received echo moves in and out of phase with the reference signal (Figure 11.12b). This results in the sample from the Doppler demodulator oscillating in magnitude at the Doppler frequency, as shown in Figure 11.12c. Often a sample and hold circuit, rather than a simple sampling gate, is used, in which case the output has the form shown by the dashed line. Since the average level of the signal from sample to sample is higher, the 'hold' has effectively given us some voltage gain.

After the signal has passed through a low-pass filter which effectively smooths the sampled (or sample-and-held) signal, we are left with the Doppler signal as shown in Figure 11.12d. As we shall see in the next section, the Doppler frequency is limited to PRF/2 and this determines the cut-off frequency of the low-pass filter.

The instrument is sensitive to flow only within a small sampling volume, which is located at a distance from the transducers such that the transit time of the transmitter pulse to the sampling volume and back again is equal to the delay between transmission and Doppler demodulator sampling. The rest of the circuit—amplifier, wall thump filter, frequency meter and loudspeaker—is the same as in the continuous wave instrument. Although one transducer is shown in the diagram it is possible to use two separate transducers for

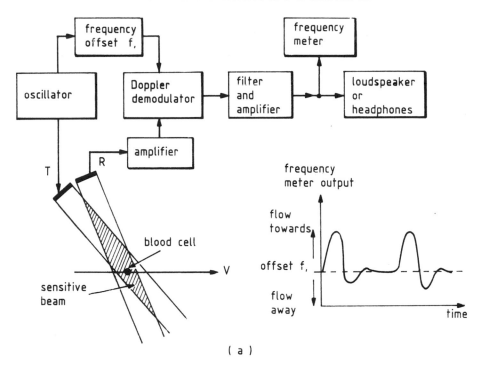

(a)

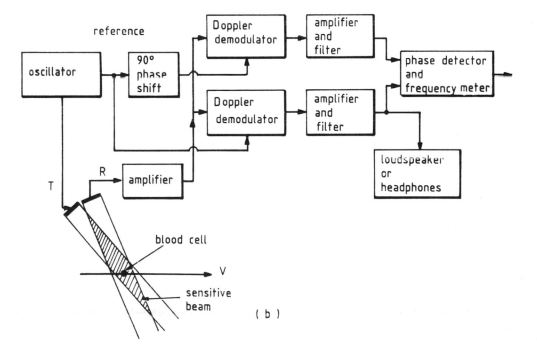

(b)

Figure 11.10 Direction discrimination by offset reference frequency (a) and by in-phase and quadrature reference signals (b).

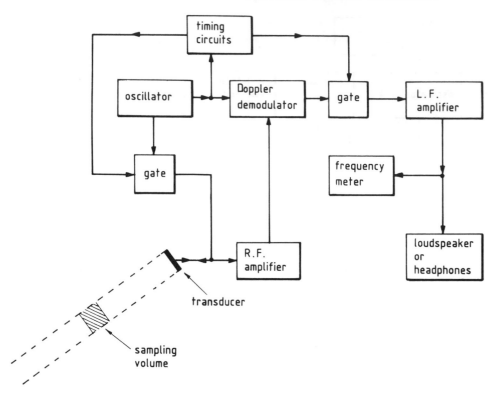

Figure 11.11 Pulsed Doppler instrument block diagram.

transmission and reception to allow switching between continuous wave and pulsed modes of operation. The length of the sample volume (which determines the axial resolution) is determined by the length of the transmitter burst and the duration of demodulator sampling. The width of the sample volume is determined by the width of the beam. The operator can examine flow at different depths by altering the transmission/sampling delay time (altering the distance of the sampling volume from the probe) and can alter the length of the sample volume by altering the duration of transmission and/or the duration of demodulator sampling. The instrument can therefore be used to look separately at vessels at different depths within the beam and also, if the sample volume is small enough, to monitor flow at different positions within a single vessel. The methods of flow direction discrimination described for use with the continuous wave

instrument may also be used with the pulsed Doppler instrument.

The instrument described is called a single-channel pulsed Doppler instrument. A multi-channel instrument, having a number of sample volumes operating simultaneously, which can monitor the flow at a number of positions along the beam at the same time, is constructed by having a number of demodulator sampling gates together with their own amplifiers and filters, each gate being opened at a different time following transmission. The potential for measuring the velocity profile in a blood vessel is illustrated in Figure 11.13.

11.5 FREQUENCY MEASUREMENT

11.5.1 Introduction

In order to measure blood velocity and monitor blood velocity waveform, it is necessary to

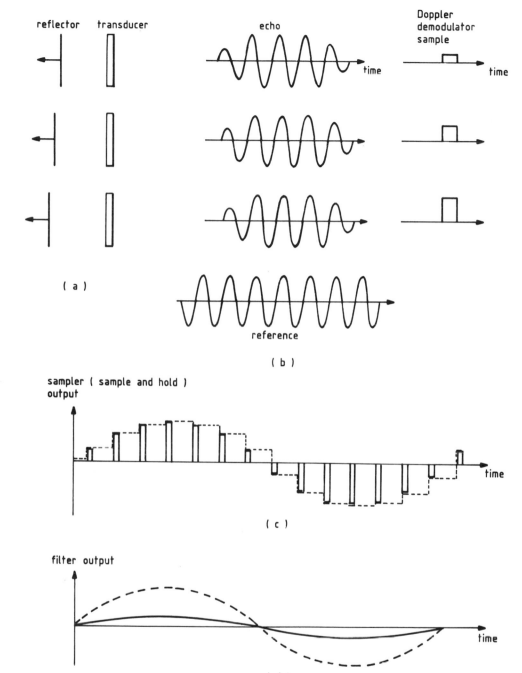

Figure 11.12 Pulsed Doppler instrument waveforms. Moving reflector/transducer geometry (a), corresponding echoes, reference signal and Doppler demodulator sample (b). Output of sampler or sample and hold circuit (c) and succeeding low-pass filter output (d). The dashed line is the filtered output of the sample and hold circuit and the solid line is the output if a simple sampler is used.

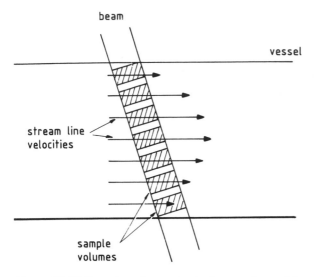

Figure 11.13 Sample volumes in the beam of a multichannel pulsed Doppler instrument, showing the potential for velocity profile measurement.

measure the Doppler shift frequency and a number of methods exist for achieving this.

11.5.2 Zero Crossing Counter

The simplest method of measurement of frequency of the Doppler signal is by the use of the zero crossing counter, which essentially counts the number of times that the signal goes through zero for a given period of time (Figure 11.14a). In practice, because the Doppler signal is inevitably mixed with background noise, thresholds are incorporated so that there is no indication on the frequency meter when only noise is present (Figure 11.17b) and the instrument counts the rate of crossing of the thresholds rather than the zero line (Figure 11.14c). The device accurately measures the frequency of a single sine wave but for a mixture of frequencies indicates the root-mean-square (RMS) frequency. In addition it gives a rather noisy output.

11.5.3 The Real-time Spectrum Analyser

A more popular method of display of the Doppler signal is on a real-time spectrum analyser. The frequency content of the Doppler signal may be shown as a graph of the amplitude of the component of the signal at a given frequency, plotted against frequency (the frequency spectrum). The spectra expected under various steady-flow conditions are shown in Figure 11.15. The spectrum for steady flow with a parabolic velocity profile and with uniform insonation of the whole vessel (Figure 11.15a) has a constant amplitude against frequency and the display is as shown with constant amplitude from the frequency corresponding to the maximum velocity down to the wall thump filter cut-off frequency. If the velocity profile is blunter, there is a concentration of signal intensity at the higher frequencies and less at the lower frequencies (Figure 11.15b). In the case of the pulsed Doppler instrument, when the range of velocities spanning the sample volume is relatively small, this is reflected as a small range of frequencies in the spectrum (Figure 11.15c). In disturbed flow at a stenosis, for example, the range of velocities and angles that the blood makes with the ultrasound beam greatly increases the range of Doppler frequencies and the spectrum becomes broadened as shown in Figure 11.15d.

In pulsatile flow conditions, the spectrum changes with time during each cardiac cycle and this variation is displayed on a real-time spectrum analyser. This instrument determines the frequency content of the signal and displays, in real-time, the amplitude of the signal at each frequency as brightness on a monitor screen (this is sometimes colour coded). The vertical axis indicates frequency and the horizontal axis time. The display axes are shown in Figure 11.16.

The display found with pulsatile flow through an artery is shown in Figure 11.17. An increase in spectral width means a decrease in the size of the systolic 'window' indicating disturbed flow.

The spectrum analysis is usually carried out using a computer which analyses a signal into

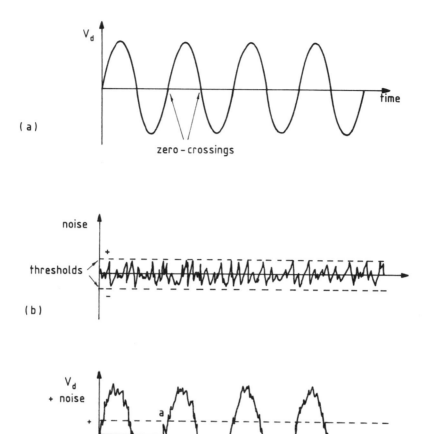

Figure 11.14 Frequency measurement by counting zero crossings. Doppler signal from a single reflector with no noise (a), noise signal with thresholds (b) and Doppler signal plus noise (c). Positive-going crossings of the positive threshold and negative-going crossings of the negative threshold are counted, e.g. at 'a' and 'b'.

frequency bands using a mathematical algorithm called the Fast Fourier Transform.

A useful waveform for analysis purposes is the maximum frequency and this can be generated on many real-time spectrum analysers by the computer detecting and drawing in the maximum frequency against time. Alternatively, analogue maximum-frequency followers are sometimes used, consisting of a narrow-band filter which tracks the edge of the frequency spectrum in time.

11.6 ALIASING

A problem which is peculiar to pulsed Doppler instruments is that of aliasing. Signals need to be sampled at least twice per cycle of their highest

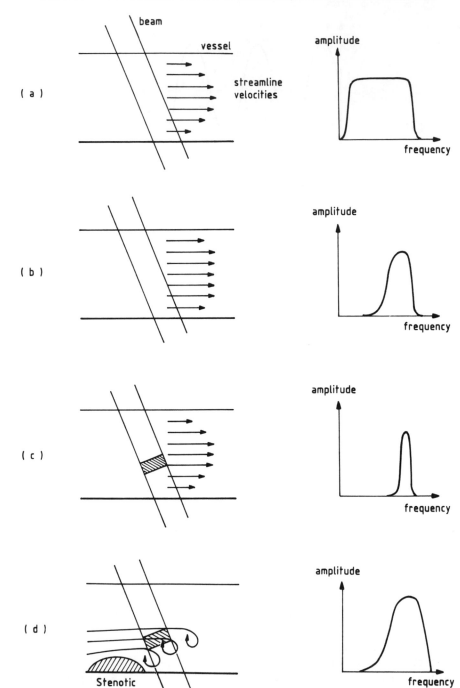

Figure 11.15 Doppler frequency spectra for various instrument and flow conditions. Continuous wave instrument with parabolic velocity profile (a), continuous wave instrument with blunt velocity profile (b), pulsed Doppler instrument with small sample volume (c) and pulsed Doppler instrument with disturbed flow (d).

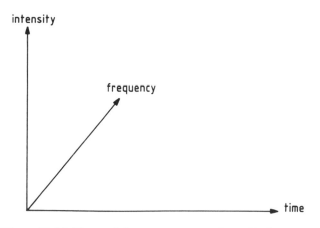

Figure 11.16 The real-time spectrum analyser display axes.

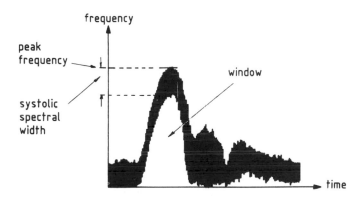

Figure 11.17 Real-time spectrum—arterial flow.

frequency component in order to unambiguously resolve that component. If the sampling frequency is too low, then the frequency of the sampled signal is in error as illustrated in Figure 11.18. In addition, in a direction-resolving pulsed Doppler instrument, the direction of flow is falsely indicated. This means that the highest Doppler shift frequency that the pulsed Doppler instrument can measure is equal to half the pulse repetition frequency of the instrument and if Doppler frequencies above this limit are present, they will be displayed as spurious frequencies equal to the Doppler shift minus the pulse reptition rate. They will appear within the limits of plus and minus half the pulse repetition frequency and changed in sign. This is illustrated in Figure 11.19.

Since the maximum repetition frequency is related to the depth of penetration, we expect this, and the maximum resolvable velocity, to be related. Since the maximum magnitude (ignoring sign) of the Doppler shift frequency is half the pulse repetition frequency (PRF) then (from equation 11.2) the magnitude of the velocity V_{max} to which this corresponds is given by:

$$\frac{PRF}{2} = \frac{2V_{max} f_0 \cos(\theta)}{c}$$

or, rearranging:

$$V_{max} = \frac{(PRF)c}{4f_0 \cos(\theta)} \qquad (11.3)$$

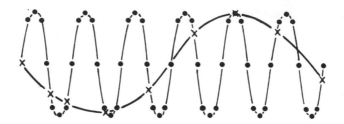

Figure 11.18 Aliasing. The shape and frequency of the sampled signal is preserved when it is sampled at a sufficiently high frequency (●). The frequency of the reconstructed signal is erroneously low when the signal is sampled at too low a frequency (×).

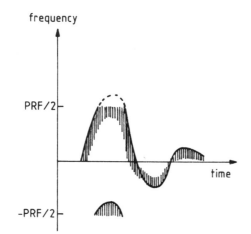

Figure 11.19 Real-time spectrum with aliasing.

From Section 5.8 we know that the maximum PRF for a maximum depth L_{max} is:

$$PRF = \frac{c}{2L_{max}}$$

Substituting in equation 11.3 and rearranging gives:

$$L_{max} V_{max} = \frac{c^2}{8f_0 \cos(\theta)} \qquad (11.4)$$

Clearly reducing the transmission frequency and increasing θ (if possible) can improve the maximum range–velocity product.

There are a number of ways of alleviating the problem of aliasing. The instrument may simply be switched from a pulsed to a continuous wave mode of operation, thereby completely removing the problem of aliasing but also removing any range resolution. Alternatively, as illustrated in Figure 11.20, the received signal may be offset in frequency before sampling, which will allow a greater frequency excursion in one direction, while reducing the range in the opposite direction. This will clearly only work if the total frequency range is less than the pulse repetition frequency. It has been proposed that the sharp change in direction at the ± PRF/2 boundaries (Figure 11.19) can be detected and the aliased portion of the waveform re-sited in its correct position on the display. This will not work if, under turbulent flow conditions, the range of Doppler frequencies (its spectral width) exceeds the pulse repetition frequency. Some manufacturers incorporate a high pulse repetition frequency mode, where the limitation on the pulse repetition

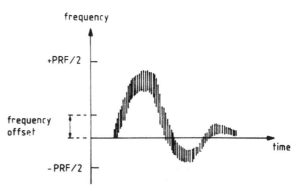

Figure 11.20 Removal of aliasing by means of a reference signal frequency offset.

frequency of the depth of penetration is simply ignored, and this leads to two or more sampling volumes operating simultaneously with the Doppler signal equal to the sum of the signals from all the sample volumes. If it is possible to arrange that only one of these sample volumes is within a vessel, then it is possible, by this method, to increase the frequency at which aliasing occurs.

11.7 CONTINUOUS WAVE/PULSED DOPPLER COMPARISON

The advantage of the pulsed Doppler instrument is that it has depth resolution and can therefore be used to monitor flow in single vessels and with small sample volumes to measure velocity variation within blood vessels. The advantages of the continuous wave Doppler instrument are that it is a simple instrument and therefore less expensive; it is easier to use since there is no depth resolution, vessels are easier to find and there is no sample volume depth and size adjustment; there is no aliasing problem; and for

a given average transmitted power the sensitivity is greater since no probe damping is required and the transducers are therefore more efficient.

11.8 DUPLEX

The Duplex system is a combination of a Doppler instrument and a real-time B-scanner. In such a system, the Doppler ultrasound beam and sample volume (in a pulsed Doppler system) are shown displayed on the B-scan image so that the beam can be directed through the vessel of interest, the sample volume can be adjusted to coincide with the B-scan image of the vessel and the operator can monitor the Doppler signals from that vessel (Figure 11.21). The system has a considerable advantage over a stand-alone Doppler system in that the flow can be monitored from selected points in the vascular tree without the difficulty of locating those points 'blind'. In addition, since the ultrasound beam and blood vessel are displayed, the angle between the vessel and the beam can be measured and the Doppler

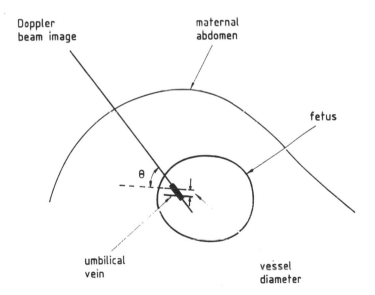

Figure 11.21 Duplex scan image—monitoring umbilical vein flow. Reproduced by permission, from Fish, P.J. (1981) Recent advances in cardio-vascular Doppler. In: A. Kurjak (ed.) *Progress in Medical Ultrasound*, Vol. 2, Elsevier.

shift frequencies translated into blood velocities.

Two transducer arrangements are used. In one arrangement the same transducer is used for B-scan and Doppler. A B-scan image is generated using the sector or linear array probe and one beam position selected to make the Doppler measurement. In the second arrangement there is a separate Doppler transducer within the B-scan transducer head and this has the advantage that the Doppler beam can be independently angled. These arrangements are illustrated in Figure 11.22. There are two modes of operation. In one the B-scan image is frozen and the Doppler sampling volume position altered with reference to the frozen image. In the second mode the frozen image is updated approximately every second using one single frame scan and during that time the Doppler information is lost.

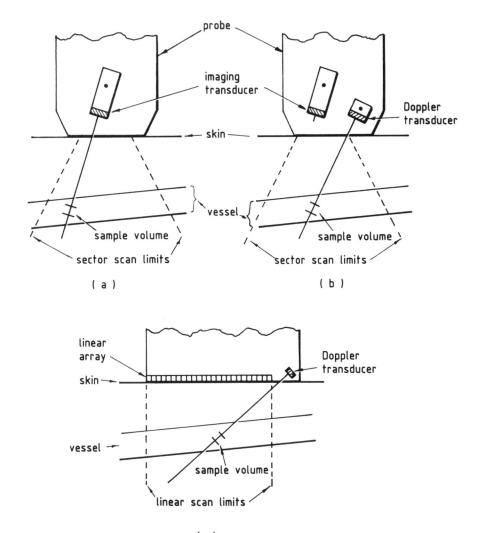

Figure 11.22 Duplex scanner probes. Mechanical sector scanner with imaging transducer used for Doppler measurements (a), mechanical scanner with separate Doppler transducer (b), and linear array with separate (fixed) Doppler transducer (c).

11.9 DOPPLER IMAGING

11.9.1 Introduction

Doppler imaging instruments are used to image the flowing blood within the vessel rather than the vessel itself.

11.9.2 The Continuous Wave Imager

The simple continuous wave Doppler imager is shown in Figure 11.23. The probe of the continuous wave Doppler instrument is attached to the arm of a position-revolving mechanism which gives an electrical output indicating the position

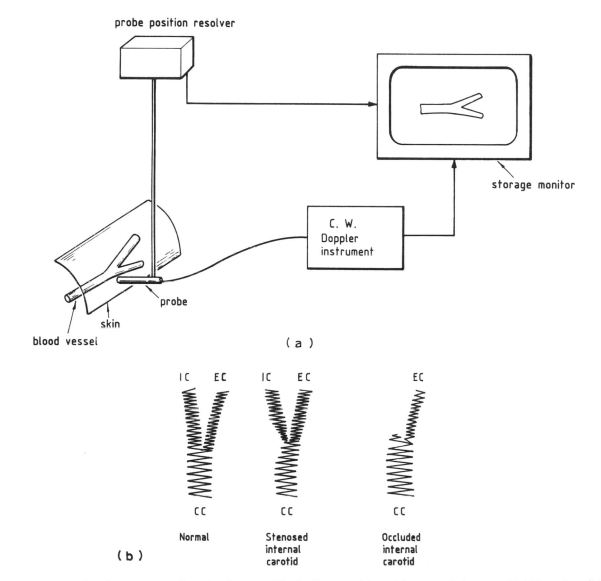

Figure 11.23 Continuous wave Doppler imager. Block diagram (a) and images of the carotid bifurcation (b) (CC, common carotid; EC, external carotid; IC, internal carotid). (a) is reproduced, by permission, from Fish, P.J. (1985) Doppler imaging. In: E. Barnett and P. Morley (eds) *Clinical Diagnostic Ultrasound*, Blackwell Scientific.

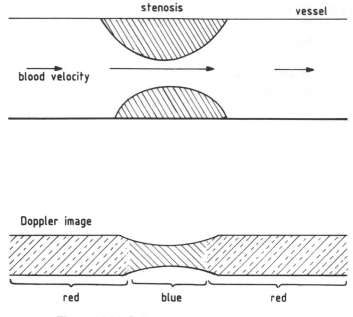

Figure 11.24 Colour coded Doppler image.

of the probe as it is moved over the skin surface. This electrical output is used to position the spot on a storage monitor and the spot is intensified and stored if the flow detector gives an output indicating that the beam is passing through a blood vessel. The image of a blood vessel (the projection of the blood vessel onto the skin surface) appears on the screen as the probe is moved in a zig-zag fashion over the vessel of interest. Complete blockages of blood vessels are shown by an absence of vessel image in the expected position and high-grade stenoses are shown as narrowing of the vessel image. The storage monitor is often replaced by a scan converter and video monitor and the image can be colour coded. This can take the form of a different colour for a different direction of flow so that normal arteries can be shown in red and veins in blue with abnormal flow reversal within a vessel being obvious. Alternatively, the measured Doppler frequency can be used to select the displayed colour, in which case the higher frequencies associated with high velocity through a stenosis can be used to indicate a stenotic region by a change of colour (Figure 11.24).

11.9.3 The Pulsed Doppler Imager

In order to generate images requiring depth information, a pulsed Doppler instrument has to be used and in this case the probe position resolver should have the three degrees of movement as shown in Figure 11.25. It is usual to use a multi-channel instrument in order to speed up the imaging process. The spots on the storage monitor now correspond to the positions of the sample volumes and the positions are calculated using the output from the position resolver and depth information from the pulsed Doppler instrument, the information being combined in the position computer. In order to generate an image of the projection of the blood vessel onto the skin surface the resolver co-ordinates ϵ and η are used to correspond to the horizontal and vertical axes of the storage monitor and the probe is moved over the skin surface in a zig-zag fashion as in the continuous wave case. In order to generate a cross-sectional image, the co-ordinates δ and η are chosen to correspond to vertical and horizontal axes and the probe is moved such that the beam passes across the blood vessel. The third

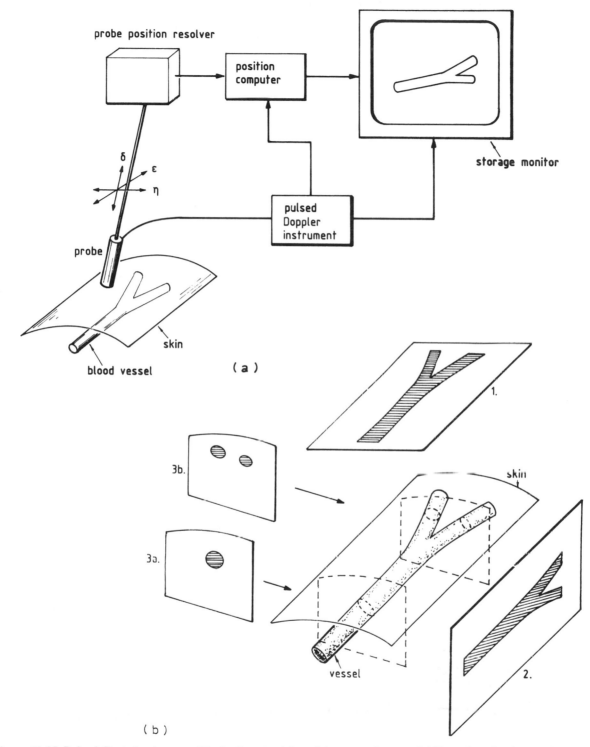

Figure 11.25 Pulsed Doppler imager. Block diagram (a) and images of a vessel bifurcation (b) (1, projection onto skin surface; 2, projection onto plane perpendicular to skin surface; 3, sectional views). (a) is reproduced by permission, from Fish, P.J. (1985) Doppler imaging. In: E. Barnett and P. Morley (eds) *Clinical Diagnostic Ultrasound*, Blackwell Scientific.

image which can be generated is the projection onto a plane perpendicular to the skin surface, in which case the resolver co-ordinates δ and ϵ are used to correspond to the vertical and horizontal axes of the storage monitor. As in the continuous wave case, a scan converter plus video monitor and colour coding may be used.

11.10 COLOURFLOW IMAGING

11.10.1 Introduction

Duplex scanners generate real-time greyscale anatomical images of vessels and allow the monitoring, using the single sample volume of the pulsed Doppler unit, of the blood velocity at selected parts of the imaged vessel. Doppler imagers, as we have seen, image the blood within the vessel as the beam is scanned by hand through the vessel of interest. These two investigation techniques are complementary and have now been combined in the colourflow imager. This device consists of a real-time B-scan imager which in addition to giving greyscale images of vessels and surrounding tissue, also detects the motion of flowing blood and displays this, in colour, within the vessel image (Figure 11.26).

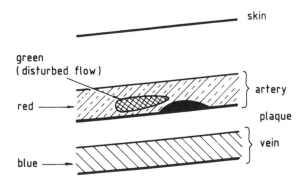

Figure 11.26 Colourflow imager display.

11.10.2 Construction

A block diagram of a colourflow imager is shown in Figure 11.27a. It should be noted that this is an essentially functional block diagram. The structure is somewhat more complex and there are considerable variations between instruments.

11.10.3 Operation

Echoes from stationary structures are the same for successive transmitted pulses along a single ultrasound beam as shown in Figure 11.27b. The stationary echo canceller simply compares the echo returns for successive transmitted pulses and removes identical signals. Thus the output from this part of the device arises solely from moving structures. As illustrated in Figure 11.27c, the received pulse from a moving reflector changes in phase from pulse to pulse, the degree of change between pulses being related to the reflector velocity. The phase detector measures this rate of change of phase and its direction and has an output related to the direction and velocity of reflector or scatterer movement at all points along the ultrasound beam. This information is sent to the scan converter and stored in the relevant part of the image store, according to beam position and reflector depth. During read-out from the scan converter to the video display, parts of the image at which motion has been detected are coloured appropriately. Normally, flow in one direction (e.g. in arteries) is coloured red and in the opposite direction (e.g. in veins) is coloured blue. Velocity can be indicated by making the colour increasingly paler as the velocity increases. Flow disturbance can be detected by the degree of variability of phase shift from pulse to pulse and this information may be stored in a similar fashion and displayed separately. For example, disturbed flow may be shown as green on the image.

This whole process can occur in parallel with normal imaging or, in some instruments, there is a periodic switch to colour imaging—using longer transmitted pulses in order to give more accurate

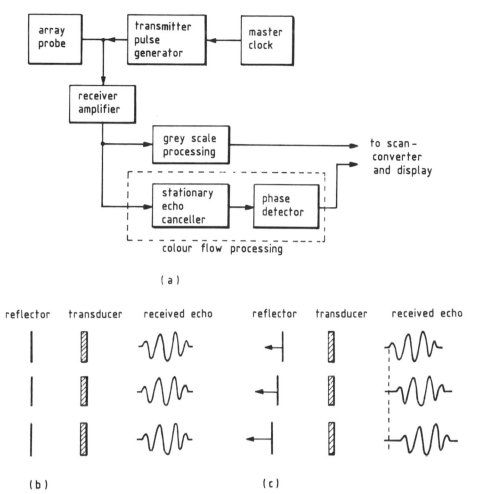

(a)

(b) (c)

Figure 11.27 Colourflow imager. Block diagram (a) and received echoes from stationary (b) and moving (c) reflectors.

measurements of the phase shifts between received pulses.

In order to reliably detect phase shift from pulse to pulse, it is necessary to average measurements over a number of transmitted pulses (of the order of 10 pulses) during which time the beam must be kept stationary in one position. There is a compromise required here. An increase in the number of pulses at each beam position leads to a greater accuracy in detecting and measuring flow and therefore to a less ragged Doppler image, but this clearly leads to a decrease

in the overall frame rate. The problem can be alleviated by choosing only a section of the B-scan image for colour coding as shown in Figure 11.28. The decrease in the number of scan lines can offset to a certain degree the larger number of pulses required for each scan line and so maintain a reasonable frame rate.

Clearly it is difficult to arrange repetitive pulses along a single scan line with a mechanical sector scanner and therefore phased and linear arrays are usually used for colourflow imaging.

As with standard Doppler devices the velocity

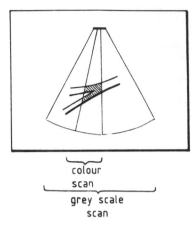

Figure 11.28 Improving frame rate by reducing colourflow image size.

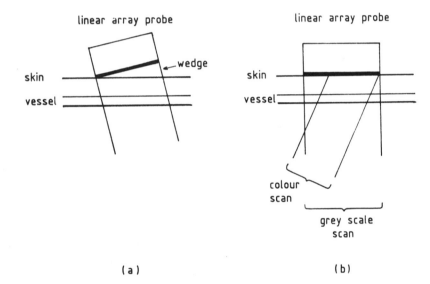

Figure 11.29 Beam angling using wedge (a) and electronic beam steering (b).

indication is dependent on beam/vessel angle and an angle other than 90° between the ultrasound beam and the blood vessel is required in order to detect motion. This can lead to some difficulty when using linear arrays on vessels which run approximately parallel to the skin surface. In this case either a wedge-shaped ultrasonic coupling device is used between the probe and the skin surface or the beams used for flow imaging are angled with respect to the B-scan image beams by electronic steering (Figure 11.29).

In order for the operator to assimilate the information contained within the image of blood flowing through a pulsatile vessel throughout a cardiac cycle, instruments may have a cine-loop type replay option in which a number of image frames are stored and replayed repetitively at a normal or slower rate. This removes the necessity to continue imaging (and therefore increasing the exposure).

CHAPTER 12

Doppler Ultrasound Measurement

12.1 INTRODUCTION

Doppler ultrasound measurements are carried out primarily to detect and measure the effect of stenoses and occlusions of blood vessels, particularly arteries.

A stenosis is shown diagrammatically in Figure 12.1a. The stenosis affects velocity, flow and pressure, creates flow disturbance and generates emboli. The stenoses form preferentially, but not exclusively, at the branches of blood vessels (e.g. the branching of the common carotid to the internal and external carotid arteries, and the aorto–iliac junction).

As a stenosis increases in severity (the residual lumen diameter decreases) there is a progressive increase in the pressure drop across the stenosis, a decrease in blood flow within the vessel and an increase in velocity within the stenosis, as shown in Figure 12.1b. Notice that it requires a high-grade stenosis (small residual lumen diameter) before there is a significant fall in blood flow—the increasing pressure drop tending to maintain the blood flow rate. There is an increase in velocity within the stenosis since the same volume of blood is passing through a smaller cross-sectional area. As the lumen size decreases, the velocity increases to a peak and then drops rapidly—reaching zero, together with the flow, at a complete occlusion. Note that the velocity within the stenosis is above normal until a very high grade stenosis is reached. A jet forms on the downstream side of high-grade stenoses and the high velocity is detectable not only within the stenosis but also for a short distance downstream until the jet dissipates in turbulent flow.

Just downstream from a stenotic lesion, the blood flow is disturbed as a result of the mixing of high-velocity blood passing the lesion and low-velocity blood immediately downstream from the lesion and close to the vessel wall (Figure 12.2).

The velocity of blood within arteries has a pulsatile nature as a result of the pumping action of the heart, and stenoses affect the velocity waveform shape as shown in Figure 12.3. The combination of the increased resistance to flow past the stenosis plus the elastic nature of the vessel wall damps the oscillation within the blood velocity pulse.

Even when the stenosis is not sufficiently severe to cause a significant reduction in blood flow, and therefore reduce oxygen and nutrient transport to tissues, the lesion can still have a severe effect by shedding parts of itself under the action of the pulsatile flow within the vessel and the periodic flexing of the vessel walls (Figure 12.4). These small particles can be sufficiently large to block or embolise smaller vessels downstream. Small areas of ischaemia may not be a severe problem in limb blood flow, but can cause temporary (transient) ischaemic attacks or stroke when present in vessels supplying the brain.

Doppler ultrasound is used to detect the presence of stenoses and measure their effect by detecting the effects mentioned above.

12.2 PRESSURE MEASUREMENT

12.2.1 Systolic Pressure

The continuous wave Doppler instrument can be used to measure systolic blood pressure in the

143

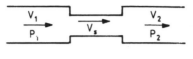

Velocity $V_1 = V_2$, $V_s > V_1$

Pressure $P_2 < P_1$

(a)

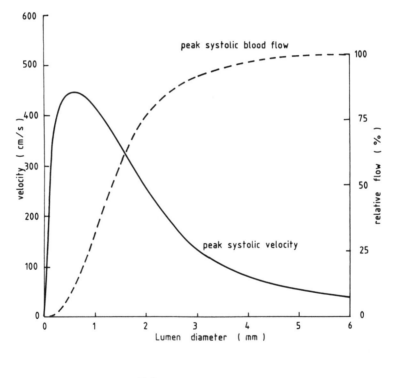

(b)

Figure 12.1 Pressure, velocity and flow rate in the vicinity of a stenosis. Pressures and velocities (a), and variation of systolic velocity and flow rate within a stenosis versus lumen diameter (b). (b) is adapted, with permission, from Spencer, M.P. (1987) *Ultrasonic Diagnosis of Cerebrovascular Disease: Doppler Techniques and Pulse Echo Imaging*, Martinus Nijhoff.

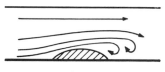

plaque

Figure 12.2 Plaque-induced flow disturbance.

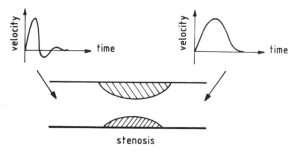

stenosis

Figure 12.3 Stenosis-induced velocity waveform change.

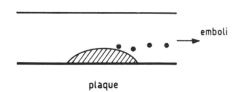

plaque

Figure 12.4 Emboli shedding from a plaque.

lower limb as indicated in Figure 12.5. Doppler signals are detected from an artery downstream from a sphygmomanometer cuff. The cuff is inflated until the artery is occluded and the Doppler signals disappear. The pressure in the cuff is then slowly released until Doppler signals are first detected. At this point, the pressure within the cuff is noted as the systolic pressure within the artery. Typical pressure measurements made at different sites on the lower limb vessels are shown in Figure 12.6, indicating the pressure drop found across a segment of vessel including a high-grade stenosis or complete occlusion of the superficial femoral artery. Note that even with a complete occlusion of a major blood vessel, the flow downstream will not normally be reduced to zero since collateral vessels, normally small, will dilate and provide a bypass of the occluded section.

12.2.2 Systolic Pressure Index

Since the measured pressure depends not only on the presence of occlusions, but also on the general systemic blood pressure, it is normal to express pressure measurements as a proportion of the brachial systolic pressure. A simple pressure index, the ratio of the systolic blood pressure at the ankle to the brachial systolic pressure, has been found to be a good indicator of disease in the vessels supplying the lower limbs. The range of values found under conditions of increasing disease severity are shown in Figure 12.7. An ankle systolic pressure index of less than one is taken to indicate disease. Pressure drops across vessel segments can be measured in order to locate the stenosis. A pressure drop of more than 30 mm of mercury across a vessel segment can be taken to indicate disease within that segment.

The effect of a stenosis can be seen more clearly if a stress test is used, for example putting the lower limb muscles in a demand state by exercise. The effect of treadmill exercise on the ankle systolic pressure index in normal subjects and patients suffering from moderate and severe claudication is shown in Figure 12.8a. The exercise is terminated after five minutes or when the patient can no longer continue, and the rate of recovery of the pressure index noted. It can be seen that little or no recovery time is required for a normal subject, a patient with moderate claudication will have recovered in six minutes whereas someone with severe claudication will still not have reached their pre-exercise index at the end of 10 minutes.

An alternative method of creating a demand state in the muscle is to occlude the supply of blood using a pressure cuff. The index measurements made before and after the five-minute occlusion are shown in Figure 12.8b. There is not such a clear distinction between

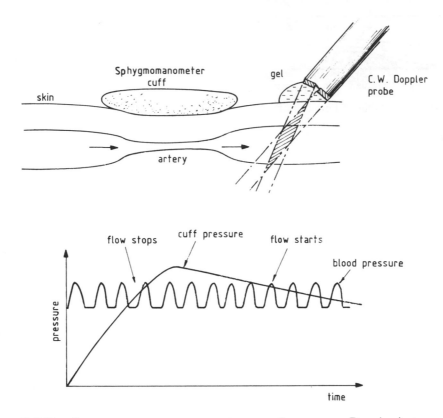

Figure 12.5 Systolic pressure measurement, using a continuous wave Doppler instrument.

normal, moderate and severe claudication in this test as with the exercise test.

12.2.3 Indirect Pressure Measurement

Obviously, non-invasive pressure measurements using sphygmomanometer cuffs cannot be used on the carotid arteries, but indirect indications of relative pressure can be found by measuring the effect on Doppler signals detected from the ophthalmic artery and its branches of a temporary compression, by finger pressure, of the superficial temporal artery. These vessels have connections both to the internal and to the external carotid arteries as shown in Figure 12.9. The pressure in the internal carotid artery is usually sufficient to give flow in these arteries in the direction shown in Figure 12.9a, whereas a high-grade stenosis in

the internal carotid artery will reverse the pressure gradient, giving the situation shown in Figure 12.9b. Compression of the superficial temple artery in normal subjects will lead to an increase in the arterial velocity, and therefore an increase in detected Doppler shift frequency, whereas in the case of an internal carotid artery stenosis, the occlusion will give rise to a diminution or reversal of flow velocity.

The pressure drop across stenosed cardiac valve orifices can be measured indirectly. With some simplifying approximations, the pressure drop (ΔP in mmHg) can be related to the velocity (v_s in ms^{-1}) in the jet from the orifice by:

$$\Delta P \simeq 4v_s^2 \qquad (12.1)$$

where v_s is calculated from the measured Doppler shift and the beam/jet angle.

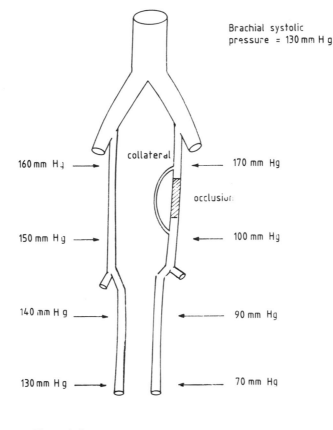

Brachial systolic
pressure = 130 mm Hg

160 mm Hg ⟶

collateral

⟵ 170 mm Hg

occlusion

150 mm Hg ⟶

⟵ 100 mm Hg

140 mm Hg ⟶

⟵ 90 mm Hg

130 mm Hg ⟶

⟵ 70 mm Hg

Ankle systolic
pressure index = 1.0   0.54

Figure 12.6 Systolic blood pressure in a healthy limb and one having an arterial occlusion. Adapted, with permission, from Atkinson, P. and Woodcock, J.P. (1982) *Doppler Ultrasound and its Use in Clinical Measurement*, p. 170. Academic Press.

12.3 VELOCITY WAVEFORM

12.3.1 Factors Affecting Waveform Shape

Two major influences on the velocity waveform are proximal stenoses, which cause a damping of the velocity waveform (Figure 12.3), and the peripheral resistance, which affects the average blood flow. Typical velocity waveforms from arteries feeding high-resistance and low-resistance vascular networks are shown in Figure 12.10. One of the noticeable characteristics of the velocity waveform in arteries feeding a low distal resistance is the relatively high end-diastolic velocity.

12.3.2 Maximum and Mean Frequency Waveforms

The velocity waveform normally used for waveform analysis is that provided by the maximum frequency or envelope of the real-time spectrum, as illustrated in Figure 12.11. This waveform reflects the variation of the maximum velocity within the vessel at any time. Note that the 'maximum' frequency envelope changes sign (indicating the most negative frequency) during the reverse flow phase. It can be appreciated that taking measurements from this waveform rather than from the mean frequency waveform gives a certain tolerance to beam or sample volume

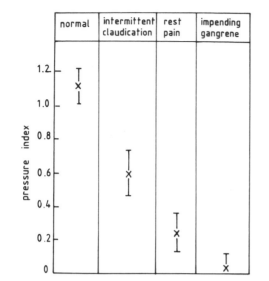

positioning and size. As long as part of the beam or sample volume passes through the area of maximum velocity, then this velocity will be registered. On the other hand, the mean frequency waveform will reflect the variation in the velocities of the stream lines passing through the beam or sample volume and will only reflect the mean velocity within the vessel if there is uniform beam or sample volume sensitivity over the whole vessel cross-section.

Figure 12.7 Ankle/brachial systolic pressure index against disease grading. Adapted, with permission, from Yao, S.T. (1970) Haemodynamic studies in peripheral disease. *British Journal of Surgery*, **57**, 761–766.

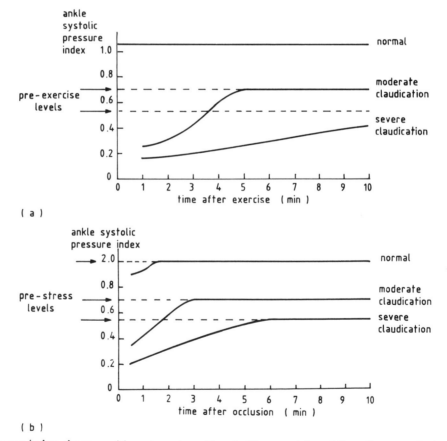

Figure 12.8 Pressure index changes with a stress test. Treadmill stress (a) and five-minute occlusion stress (b). Reproduced, with permission, from Baker, J.D. (1982) Stress testing. In: R.F. Kempczinski and J.S.T. Yao (eds) *Practical Noninvasive Vascular Diagnosis*, Year Book Medical Publishers.

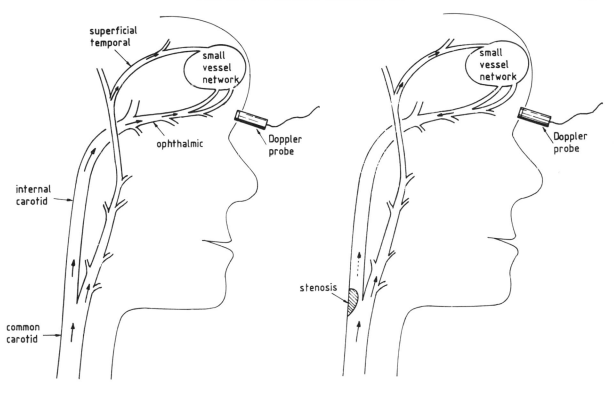

Figure 12.9 Ophthalmic artery flow in normal subject (a) and with stenosed internal carotid artery (b). Adapted, with permission, from Moore, W.S. and Barton, A.B. (1982) Periorbital Doppler examination (ophthalmosonometry) and supraorbital photoplethysmography. In: R.F. Kempczinski and J.S.T. Yao (eds) *Practical Noninvasive Vascular Diagnosis*, Year Book Medical Publishers.

12.3.3 Waveform Indices—Introduction

Indices of velocity waveform shape as opposed to absolute velocity measurements are attractive because they are largely independent of the angle between the ultrasound beam and the blood vessel. Although, as shown in Figure 12.12, the absolute magnitude of the Doppler frequency waveform changes with this angle, the shape of the waveform remains unchanged.

Simple indices of waveform shape which have been used to detect vessel disease are shown in Figure 12.13.

12.3.4 The Pulsatility Index

The pulsability index (PI) is a good indicator of waveform damping, due to stenoses in the vessels supplying the lower limbs—a low PI indicates a high degree of damping.

12.3.5 The Pourcelot Index

The Pourcelot index is an indicator of peripheral resistance, the index increasing as the end-diastolic velocity decreases, indicating increasing

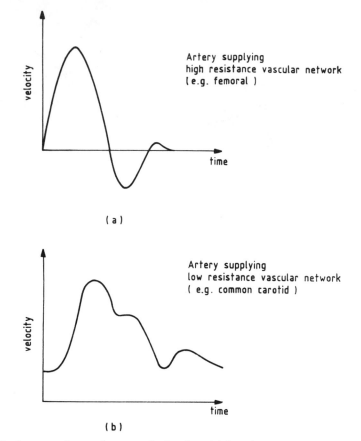

(a)

(b)

Figure 12.10 Typical velocity waveforms for vessels feeding high-resistance vascular network (a) and low-resistance network (b).

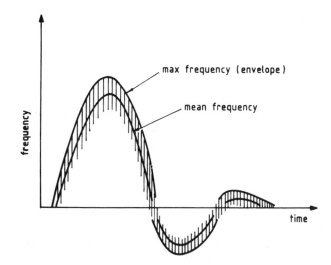

Figure 12.11 Real-time spectrum showing the maximum frequency and mean frequency curves.

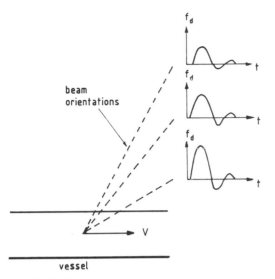

Figure 12.12 Doppler frequency waveform for various beam/vessel angles. Reproduced, with permission, from Johnson, K.W. *et al.* (1981) Real-time frequency analysis of peripheral arterial Doppler signals. In: E.B. Diethrich (ed.) *Noninvasive Vascular Diagnosis*, 2nd Edition, p. 236. PSG Publishing.

peripheral resistance. The normal range for the common carotid artery waveform shown is 0.55–0.75. Higher values indicate disease.

12.3.6 The A/B Ratio

The A/B ratio used for carotid artery disease is a somewhat more empirical index. It is found that in diseased vessels, the height of the plateau or second peak (B) is the common carotid artery waveform increases relative to the main systolic peak velocity (A), so reducing the A/B ratio. Disease is indicated if the ratio is less than 1.05.

12.3.7 Laplace Transform Analysis

A more complex analysis of velocity waveform shape is that of Laplace Transform Analysis. As shown in Figure 12.14 this form of analysis matches the measured waveform to the sum of a damped oscillation and an exponential decay. The analysis provides three quantities (ω_0, γ, δ).

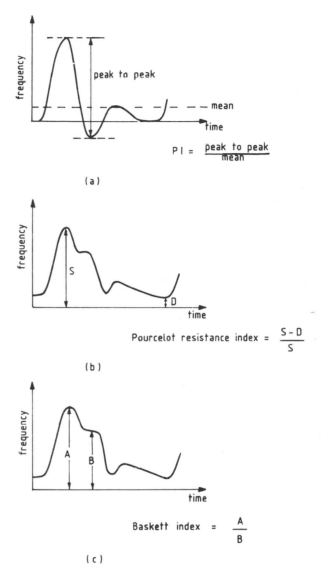

Figure 12.13 Indices of velocity waveform shape. Pulsatility index (a), Pourcelot resistance index (b) and Baskett index (c).

The first (ω_0) is proportional to the frequency of oscillation of the damped oscillatory part of the waveform. This is governed by the vessel elasticity. Secondly, the rate of decay (γ) of the exponential part of the waveform is governed by the peripheral resistance. It has been found that the most useful quantity to be given by this analysis is the Laplace transform damping factor

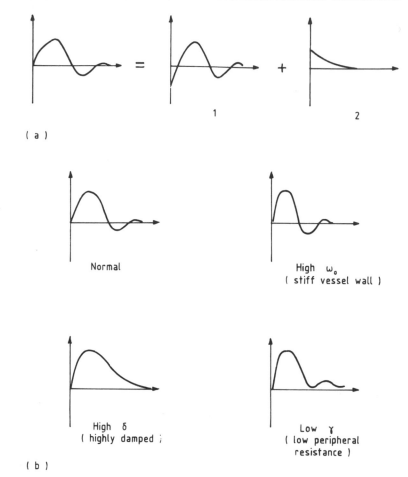

Figure 12.14 Laplace analysis. Velocity waveform as the sum of a damped sine wave and an exponential curve (a) and velocity waveforms for various disease conditions (b).

(δ), which is the measure of the degree of damping of the oscillatory part of the waveform. This is related to proximal stenosis but is also affected by peripheral resistance.

12.3.8 Principal Component Analysis

Another complex method of waveform analysis is called Principal Component Analysis. We have seen, when considering the spectrum of the transmitted ultrasound pulse, that a waveform can be considered as the sum of a series of other waveforms. In that case, we considered a series of sine waves of different frequencies as the components of the pulse. Other waveform series can be used in this way. The only constraint is that the series is orthogonal, which is to say that any one waveform of the series cannot, itself, be described by a sum of any of the others. The principal components of, for example, the femoral artery waveform, are those orthogonal waveforms a sum of which can be used to describe the femoral artery waveform with the minimum number of components. The principal component waveforms for the femoral artery waveform are

Principal components

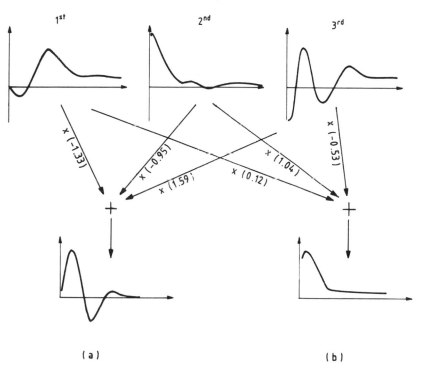

(a)   (b)

Figure 12.15 Principal component analysis. The normal (a) and abnormal (b) femoral artery waveforms are shown as the sum of different proportions of the principal components of a set of femoral artery waveforms. Adapted, with permission, from Walton, L. *et al.* (1983) An objective feature extraction technique. In: R.A. Lerski and P. Morley (eds) *Ultrasound '82*, p. 265. © 1983 Pergamon Press PLC.

shown in Figure 12.15. Normal and abnormal velocity waveforms are shown as a sum of different fractions of these components. The coefficients (multiplying factors) of the principal components for any one velocity waveform measurement are used to indicate whether that waveform is normal or abnormal.

12.3.9 Damping Factor and Inverse Damping Factor

The degree of damping of a waveform over a particular section of blood vessel can be calculated from measurements made of the pulsatility index at the beginning and end of that segment, and the damping factor (DF) is then given by:

$$DF = \text{Proximal PI} \div \text{Distal PI} \qquad (12.2)$$

Some people have used the inverse damping factor:

$$DF^{-1} = \text{Distal PI} \div \text{Proximal PI} \qquad (12.3)$$

A high value of damping factor or low value of inverse damping factor indicates a stenosis or occlusion in that segment of vessel, as illustrated in Figure 12.16.

Typical pulsatility indices and inverse damping factors for aorto-iliac, superficial femoral and mixed disease are shown in Figure 12.17. Figure 12.18 shows the normal ranges for PI and inverse damping factor for various grades of stenoses.

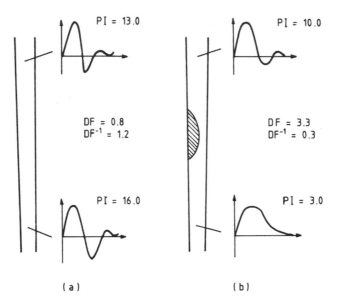

Figure 12.16 Pulsatility index, damping factor and inverse damping factor for normal (a) and stenosed (b) lower limb artery segments.

12.3.10 Pulse Transit Time

The velocity at which a pressure pulse and its accompanying velocity wave travel down an artery is a function of the elasticity of the vessel wall. A stiff-walled vessel will have a high pulse-wave velocity. The transit time of the pressure pulse from one part of the vessel to another is used diagnostically as indicated in Figure 12.19. A high value of transit time indicates a complete occlusion of the main vessel with the pressure pulse travelling a longer distance through collateral vessels. A shorter than normal transit time indicates generalised but non-occluding disease of the main vessel leading to a stiffening of the arterial wall. A damped waveform, together with a normal transit time, indicates a non-occluding lesion of the main vessel. The transit times are measured using two continuous wave Doppler instruments at the beginning and end of the vessel segment under investigation, the velocity waveforms from each being passed to a single chart recorder from which the transit time can be measured as shown in Figure 12.20. Alternatively, the transit time can be measured automatically from the two waveforms.

12.3.11 Normalised Transit Time and Damping Factor

It is found that a better separation of normal and diseased vessels can be made if the transit time and the damping factor over a vessel cross-section are 'normalised', that is to say each divided by the average transit time and damping factor found in a group of normal subjects of the same age range as the patient. This procedure eliminates the effect of normal changes of transit time and damping factor with age. Figure 12.21 indicates the normal and diseased-state ranges of the normalised transit time and damping factors.

12.4 SPECTRAL ANALYSIS

Spectral analysis, as indicated in Figure 12.22, can be used to detect the presence of stenotic lesions by indicating the increase in velocity in

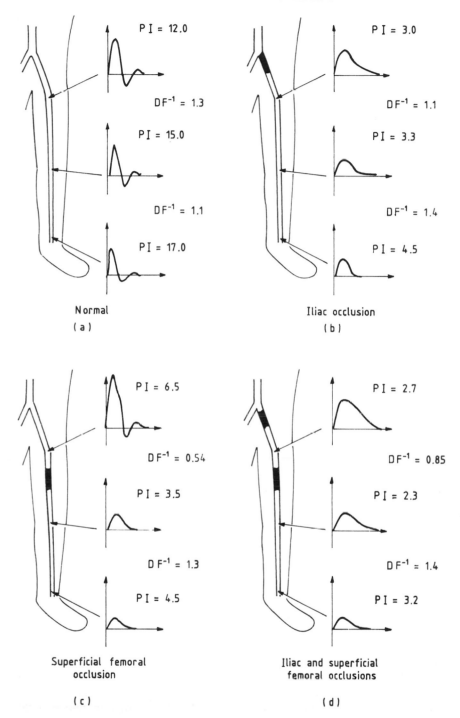

Figure 12.17 Pulsatility indices and inverse damping factors in lower limb vessels for various disease states. Adapted, with permission, from *Ultrasound in Medicine and Biology*, **4(3)**, Johnston, K.W. *et al.* © 1978 Pergamon Press PLC.

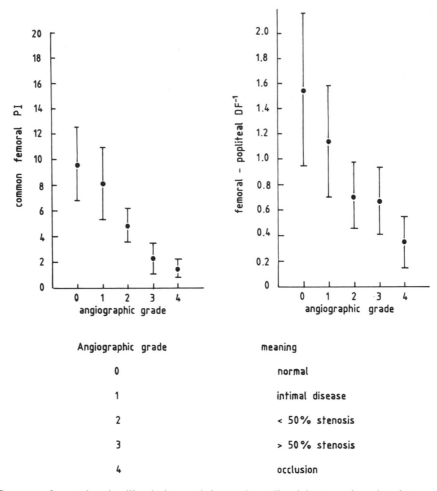

Angiographic grade	meaning
0	normal
1	intimal disease
2	< 50% stenosis
3	> 50% stenosis
4	occlusion

Figure 12.18 Common femoral pulsatility index and femoral–popliteal inverse damping factor versus grade of stenosis. Reproduced, with permission, from *Ultrasound in Medicine and Biology*, **4(3)**, Johnston, K.W. *et al.* © 1978 Pergamon Press PLC.

the jet through a stenosis, together with the spectral broadening (increase in the range of Doppler shift frequencies) resulting from an increase in the range of velocities and the range of angles between beam and direction of flow in the region of disturbed flow. It is usual to use a pulsed Doppler instrument (usually part of a Duplex scanner) rather than a continuous wave instrument since the spectrum in the normal vessel is broader when using a continuous wave instrument as we have seen in Figure 11.15. For the same reason it is usual to use a small sample volume when using the pulsed Doppler instrument.

Since the Doppler signal arises from the passage of a random collection of blood cells passing through the beam or sample volume, the Doppler signal itself has a random nature. Since the spectrum at different times in the cardiac cycle is estimated from short time segments (2–20 ms) of the Doppler signal, the measured spectrum for one cardiac cycle is very irregular. In order to make a measurement of spectral width to aid in the discrimination between different degrees of stenosis, the spectra measured at similar points in a number of cardiac cycles may be averaged as shown in Figure 12.23 in order to achieve a more accurate measurement of spectral width.

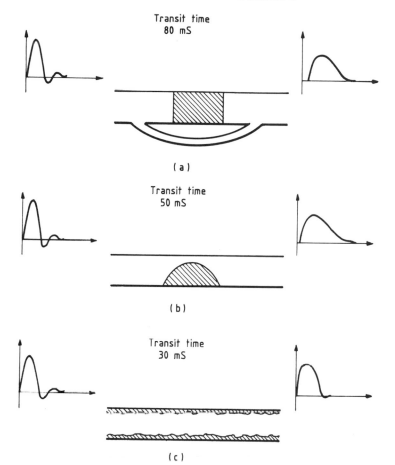

Figure 12.19 Waveform changes and transit times for various disease states in the common femoral to popliteal artery segment. Complete occlusion bypassed by collaterals (a), non-occluding lesion (b) and generalised disease (c). Adapted, with permission, from Atkinson, P. and Woodcock, J.P. (1982) *Doppler Ultrasound and its Use in Clinical Measurement*, p. 182. Academic Press.

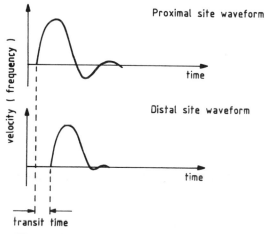

Figure 12.20 Measurement of transit time.

Suitable spectral broadening indices (SBI) are:

$$\text{SBI}_1 = f_{max} \div f_{mean} \qquad (12.4)$$

or

$$\text{SBI}_2 = (f_{max} - f_{min}) \div f_{mean} \qquad (12.5)$$

both of which will increase as flow disturbance increases the spectral width.

Tables 12.1 and 12.2 show the Doppler spectrum characteristics for various grades of stenoses in the lower limb vessels and carotid arteries respectively.

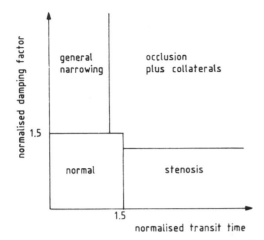

Figure 12.21 Disease categorisation using normalised damping factors and transit times. Adapted, with permission, from Gosling, R.G. (1976) Extraction of physiological information from spectrum-analysed Doppler-shifted continuous-wave ultrasound signals obtained non-invasively from the arterial system. In: D.W. Hill and B.W. Watson (eds) *IEEE Medical Electronics Monographs 18–22*, Institution of Electrical Engineers.

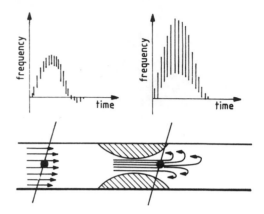

Figure 12.22 Real-time spectrum changes downstream from a stenosis.

Table 12.1 Spectra from Duplex scans of lower limb vessels.

Angiographic findings (diameter stenosis)	Doppler spectrum
Normal	Tri- or bi-phasic waveform. No broadening.
1–19%	Normal waveform. Small degree of spectral broadening.
20–49%	30–50% increase in peak systolic velocity. Reverse component present. Spectral broadening.
50–99%	50–100% increase in peak systolic velocity. High degree of spectral broadening. Highly damped waveform (no reverse component).
Occluded	No Doppler signal at site.

Reproduced from Neumyer, M.M. and Thiel, B.L. (1988) Evaluation of lower extremity occlusive disease with Doppler ultrasound. In: K. Taylor *et al.* (ed.) *Clinical Applications of Doppler Ultrasound*, p. 332. Raven Press.

Table 12.2 Spectra from Duplex scans of carotid arteries.

Angiographic findings (diameter stenosis)	Doppler spectrum
Normal	$V_s \leq 125$ cm/s or $f_s \leq 4$ kHz.
1–15%	$V_s \leq 125$ cm/s or $f_s \leq 4$ kHz. Small degree of spectral broadening on decelerative phase of systole.
16–49%	$V_s \leq 125$ cm/s or $f_s \leq 4$ kHz. Broadening during the whole of systole. (No systolic 'window'.)
50–99%	$V_s > 125$ cm/s or $f_s > 4$ kHz. Broadening during the whole of systole.
Occlusion	No Doppler signal from ICA. Zero end-diastolic velocity in CCA.

Transmitted frequency = 5 MHz, beam/vessel angle = 60°. (V_s = indicated peak systolic velocity, f_s = peak systolic Doppler shift frequency).

Reprinted with permission from *Ultrasound in Medicine and Biology*, **9**, Langlois, Y. *et al.* Evaluating carotid artery disease. © 1983, Pergamon Press PLC.

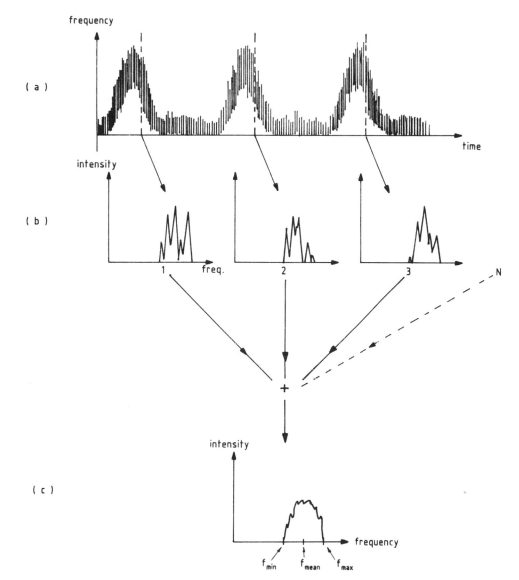

Figure 12.23 Frequency spectrum averaging. The frequency spectra of the Doppler signals taken at similar points in N consecutive cardiac cycles are averaged to arrive at a less noisy spectrum on which spectral width measurements can be made. Real-time spectrum (a), individual spectra (b) and average spectrum (c).

12.5 BEAM/VESSEL ANGLE AND VELOCITY MEASUREMENT

12.5.1 Methods

In order to convert measured Doppler shift frequencies to velocity a measurement of the angle between the ultrasound beam and the blood vessel is required. From equation 11.2:

$$V = \frac{-f_d c}{2f_0 \cos(\theta)} \qquad (12.6)$$

There are a number of ways that this can be achieved. The Doppler probe can be moved such that the beam remains within the blood vessel but the Doppler shift frequency drops to zero, in which case the beam is known to be perpendicular to the blood vessel and can be moved through a measured angle. Two Doppler transducers can be mounted in the same probe at an angle as shown in Figure 12.24. If the orientation of this probe is altered such that the Doppler frequency from one transducer is equal in magnitude but opposite in sign to that from the other transducer then it is known that the probe body is parallel to the blood vessel and the angles of the two beams to the vessel are equal.

The most widely used method of angle measurement has already been mentioned. Using a Duplex scanner the vessel image and beam are visible simultaneously on the screen and the angle can be measured directly. In most Duplex instruments an electronically generated line passing through the sample volume image can be rotated until it is parallel to the vessel axis and the instrument then knows the orientation of the vessel with respect to the beam and can automatically calculate velocities from measured Doppler shift frequencies (Figure 12.25).

12.5.2 Errors

Errors in the measurement of frequency and beam vessel angle will affect the accuracy of velocity calculation. Errors in the measured frequency are caused by poor signal level such that the background noise has a significant effect on the measured frequency, or the signal is below thresholds set in order to reject background noise. There is a random error resulting from the random nature of the Doppler signal and from physiological variations, which may be alleviated by averaging over a number of cardiac cycles. The 'wall thump' filter used to remove low-frequency Doppler signals arising from tissue movement will also remove low-frequency Doppler signals from slowly moving blood so that the signals with these frequencies will not be present in any mean frequency estimation, leading to an overestimation of mean frequency.

The angle measurement may be in error as a

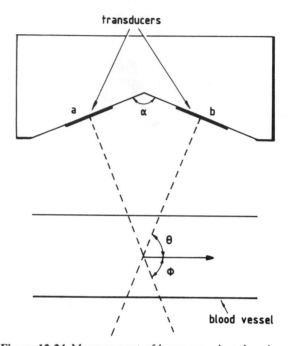

Figure 12.24 Measurement of beam vessel angle using a two-transducer pulsed Doppler probe. When correctly adjusted, $\theta = \psi = \alpha/2$. Reproduced, with permission, from Fish, P.J. (1982) Recent advances in cardiovascular Doppler. In: A. Kurjak (ed.) *Progress in Medical Ultrasound*, Elsevier.

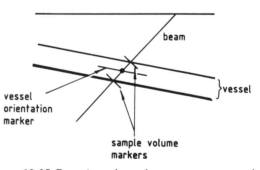

Figure 12.25 Beam/vessel angle measurement using electronic vessel orientation marker.

result of misalignment of the vessel axis marker, by the ultrasound beam from a probe being at an angle to the probe axis and from refraction of the ultrasound beam in tissue.

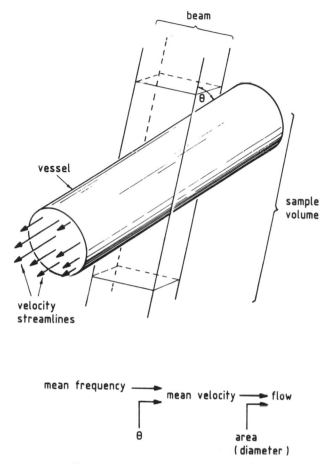

Figure 12.26 Flow measurement—uniform sensitivity method. Adapted, with permission, from Fish P.J. (1982) Recent advances in cardio-vascular Doppler. In: A. Kurjak (ed.) *Progress in Medical Ultrasound*, Elsevier.

12.6 FLOW MEASUREMENT

12.6.1 Introduction

Measurements of blood flow are of use in assessing the rate of supply of oxygen to organs. There are basically two methods of flow measurement.

12.6.2 The Uniform Sensitivity Method

This method is by far the most common. It is illustrated in Figure 12.26. The sample volume is made to span the vessel of interest. The instru-

ment calculates the mean Doppler shift frequency, which can be used to calculate mean velocity when the beam/vessel angle is used. Since flow equals velocity multiplied by cross-sectional area, a measurement of vessel cross-sectional area (usually using a measurement of diameter using electronic calipers on the Duplex scanner and assuming a circular cross-section vessel) can be used by the instrument to convert mean velocity to a volume flow rate.

12.6.3 The Velocity Profile Method

This method is illustrated in Figure 12.27. The

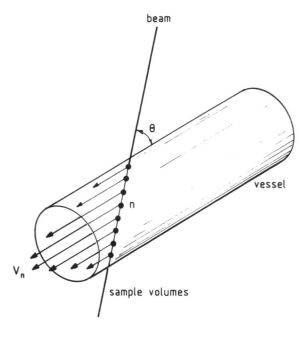

beam

θ

n

V_n

vessel

sample volumes

frequency profile ——▶velocity profile ——▶ flow

θ

Figure 12.27 Flow measurement—velocity profile method. Adapted, with permission, from Fish, P.J. (1982) Recent advances in cardio-vascular Doppler. In: A. Kurjak (ed.) *Progress in Medical Ultrasound*, Elsevier.

angle is measured as before, the variation in blood velocity is measured, using a multi-channel instrument, across the blood vessel diameter and, assuming axially symmetric flow, the flow can be calculated by adding up the contributions of all the velocity stream lines within the vessel cross-section.

12.6.4 Errors

The errors in flow measurement arise from the errors in velocity measurement described in Section 12.5.2 and errors peculiar to the particular method of flow measurement. There will be an error in flow measurement using the uniform sensitivity method if the sensitivity of the instrument is not uniform over the whole vessel cross-section, leading to an error in mean velocity. This can arise quite easily, since pulsed Doppler instruments normally have the facility to increase the sample volume length but not its width (beam width) so that it is not always possible to guarantee uniform sensitivity over a range of vessel sizes. Usually the dominant error in this method of flow measurement is that arising from the cross-sectional area measurement. Firstly, the cross-sectional area will change during the cardiac cycle as a result of the pulsatile nature of the blood pressure and the elastic nature of the vessel walls. Strictly speaking the flow should be calculated at intervals during the cardiac cycle by multiplying instantaneous velocity by instantaneous cross-sectional area. In practice it is usual to measure an average cross-sectional area and use this figure. The errors arising from the cross-sectional area measurement, particularly via a measurement of diameter, were discussed in Chapter 10.

The velocity profile method also suffers from inaccuracies due to the finite size of the sample volumes which mean that the velocity profile cannot be accurately measured, particularly near the vessel walls, and the assumption that the velocity profile over the whole vessel cross-section is axially symmetric.

12.7 SOME OTHER PRECAUTIONS AND ARTIFACTS

12.7.1 Standard Conditions

Since the peripheral impedance is altered by muscle demand state, it is important that patients rest for at least 20 minutes before measurements are made, in order to establish standard conditions for the measurements. In addition, limb temperatures will affect blood flow, superficial vessels being constricted and therefore increasing peripheral resistance at low temperatures and becoming dilated in order to provide cooling at higher temperatures. Ideally, measurements should be carried out in a constant-temperature room.

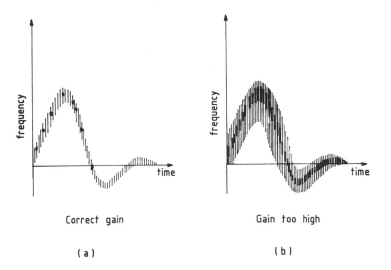

Figure 12.28 Spurious Doppler spectral broadening resulting from analyser overload.

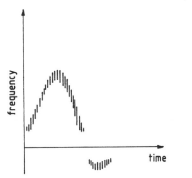

Figure 12.29 Waveform distortion due to wall thump filter artifact.

12.7.2 Spectrum Overload

It is important when making spectrum measurements to reduce the gain of the Doppler system to the point where peak intensity is only reached occasionally in the displayed spectrum. Increasing the Doppler signal level will give rise to spurious indications of spectral broadening due to overload of the spectral analysis circuit, as illustrated in Figure 12.28.

12.7.3 Wall Thump Filter Artifact

As we have seen before, the 'wall thump' filter removes not only those low Doppler frequency signals arising from vessel wall movement, but also the low Doppler frequency signals arising from slowly moving blood. The cut-off frequency of the filter is often adjustable and setting this too high can remove diastolic flow signals and give an erroneous indication of velocity pulsatility or end-diastolic flow velocity (Figure 12.29).

12.8 CALIBRATION

Some test rigs which can be used for checking the calibration of Doppler instruments are shown in Figure 12.30. The accuracy of velocity measurement using a Doppler instrument can be checked by pointing the ultrasound probe towards a motor-driven reflector (Figure 12.30a) moving at a known speed and noting the difference between measured and expected Doppler frequency. A motor-driven continuous loop of string (Figure 12.30b) can be used to simulate a velocity stream line. In this case the probe can be checked at a

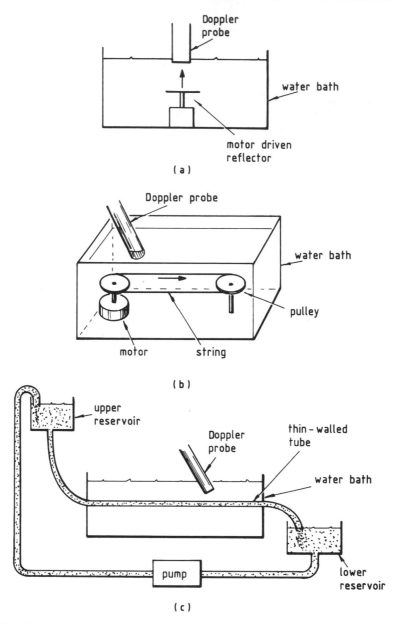

Figure 12.30 Doppler instrument test rigs. Moving reflector (a), moving string (b), and flow rig (c).

number of angles to the velocity direction. A fluid containing scattering particles such as small plastic beads (Figure 12.30c) can be made to flow through a thin-walled plastic or rubber tube within a water bath and the fluid velocity calculated from the flow rate measured using a measuring cylinder and stopwatch. If the flow is steady and there is a sufficiently long length of tube before the measurement site, the velocity profile can be assumed to be parabolic, in which case the maximum velocity is twice the mean velocity. The flow rate can also be used to check the accuracy of flow measurements using a Doppler instrument.

CHAPTER 13

Digital Storage, Scan Converters and Data Processing

13.1 INTRODUCTION

In order to store, temporarily, ultrasound or Doppler signal data in a form which will allow us to process it in order to gain more information than is immediately apparent, we need to make use of digital number storage and computer techniques.

13.2 BINARY ARITHMETIC

Computers store and perform calculations using numbers in a binary representation.

In the conventional representation of numbers, each digit in the number can have one of ten values from 0 to 9 and each digit represents a different power of 10. In binary numbers each digit can have one of two values, either 0 or 1, and each digit represents a different power of 2.

The number 429, for example, can be represented in the decimal system as:

Digit	4	2	9
Factor	10^2	10	1

and the binary system as:

Digit	1	1	0	1	0	1	1	0	1
Factor	2^8	2^7	2^6	2^5	2^4	2^3	2^2	2	1

Binary digits are usually called bits and the digit on the extreme left is the most significant bit (MSB) and the digit on the extreme right the least significant bit (LSB).

The binary system allows numbers to be stored in devices having two states. For example, the store could be a number of capacitors, charged representing a 1 and uncharged representing a 0, in a magnetic medium, magnetisation in one direction representing 0 and magnetisation in the other direction representing 1, and electronic switches, with their 'on' and 'off' states representing 0 and 1.

The maximum number of bits available to store each number limits the maximum number that can be stored. For example, the maximum numbers that can be stored in 4 and 8 bits are 15 and 255 respectively as shown below.

4-bit number:

Factor	8	4	2	1		
Min. =	0	0	0	0	=	0
Max. =	1	1	1	1	=	15

8-bit number:

Factor	128	64	32	16	8	4	2	1		
Min.	0	0	0	0	0	0	0	0	−	0
Max.	1	1	1	1	1	1	1	1	=	255

Computers usually use binary numbers in multiples of 8 bits. The group of 8 bits is called a byte and the number in 1, 2 or 4 bytes (8, 16 or 32 bits) is called a word.

13.3 COMPUTERS

Computers are used to perform calculations on numbers presented to them from various devices, to display on output devices and to store information for later analysis. A block diagram is shown in Figure 13.1. The central processor unit (CPU) is the organising part of the instrument.

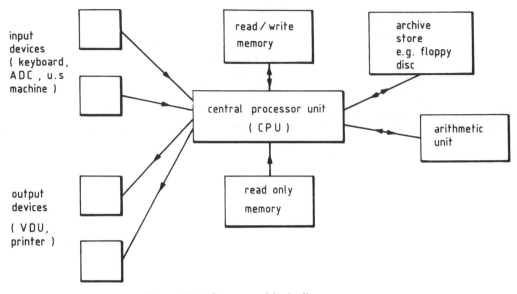

Figure 13.1 Computer block diagram.

It operates according to a sequence of instructions (the program) stored in one of the memory units. The read-only memory (ROM) can contain permanent programs and data, and the read/write or random access memory (RAM) and the magnetic disc memory can hold programs and data on a temporary basis. Information can be read from or written to the read/write memory rapidly, whereas the disc is a somewhat slower storage medium but often larger.

The disc can be rigid (a 'hard' disc) and usually permanently installed within the instrument, or a lower capacity and removable 'floppy' disc.

Numbers may be input from the keyboard or from an analogue to digital converter (described later) or directly in digital format from an ultrasound machine. Calculations are performed, making use of the arithmetic unit, and results displayed on a visual display unit, ultrasound machine screen or printer and, if necessary, stored for later analysis on floppy disc.

13.4 MEMORY

Numbers and instructions coded as numbers are stored in binary format on electronic switches,

capacitors or magnetic media in a form which is shown diagrammatically in Figure 13.2. Each number has a numerical address by which the computer can find the number (e.g. 54). Thus, to find the number stored at location X in the diagram, the computer would switch on the address lines intersecting at the point X as shown. The memory would then output, on the data lines, the number stored at this location.

13.5 THE MAGNETIC DISC

This store consists of a disc coated with a magnetic material rotating at high speed within a disc drive unit (Figure 13.3). Binary information is written to and read from the disc by a small electromagnet which will create a small magnet on the disc surface underneath it when energised. The direction of current through the coil of the electromagnet will determine the orientation of the magnet created on the disc surface and therefore determine whether a 0 or 1 is written. The same electromagnet is used to read the data on the disc, in which case the small magnet on the surface of the disc will give rise to voltages of different directions representing 0s or 1s. The

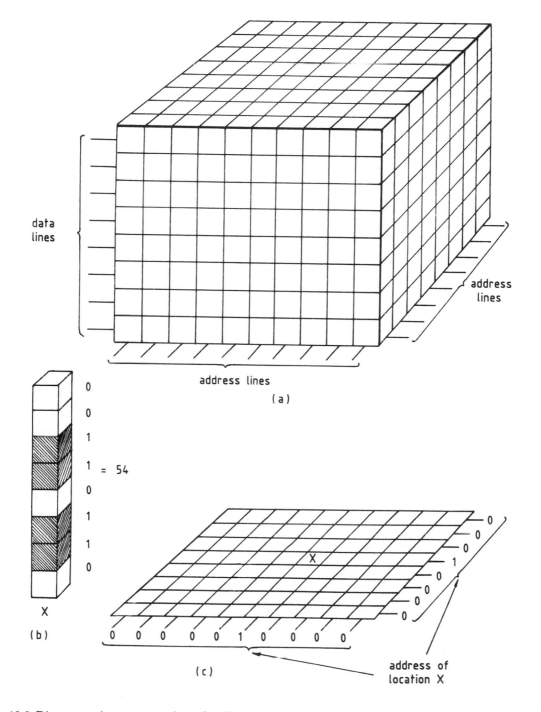

Figure 13.2 Diagrammatic representation of a digital memory (a). The location of a particular number (b) in memory is given by its position in the horizontal plane (c) and the numbers are stored vertically as binary digits.

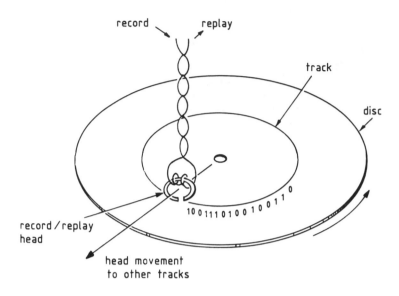

Figure 13.3 Magnetic disc store.

electromagnet is moved radially across the disc surface in order to write numbers on different tracks.

13.6 THE ANALOGUE TO DIGITAL CONVERTER (ADC)

It is frequently required to store a continually varying (analogue) signal, such as an A-scan, in digital format. The device which performs the conversion is called the analogue to digital converter (ADC).

This device is illustrated in Figure 13.4. It samples an analogue signal at regular intervals and converts the level of the signal at each sampling time into a proportional number in binary format. In the example shown, if a 10-V input is represented by the number 256 then the sample of 2.1 V is represented by the number 54. Clearly the sampling should be sufficiently frequent to follow the most rapid change of the analogue signal.

13.7 THE DIGITAL TO ANALOGUE CONVERTER (DAC)

This is the opposite process, converting from numbers in a binary format to an analogue voltage, and is illustrated in Figure 13.5.

13.8 SCAN CONVERTERS (see also Section 6.5)

13.8.1 Introduction

This device, based on a digital store or memory, is used to convert the format of the echo information from the ultrasound scanner into a form suitable for display on a video monitor. The scan plane is divided up into a rectangular grid as shown in Figure 13.6, each square representing a small area of tissue, having a corresponding address in the (image) memory and a small area for display (pixel) on the monitor. Thus, an echo arriving from the position marked x will have a

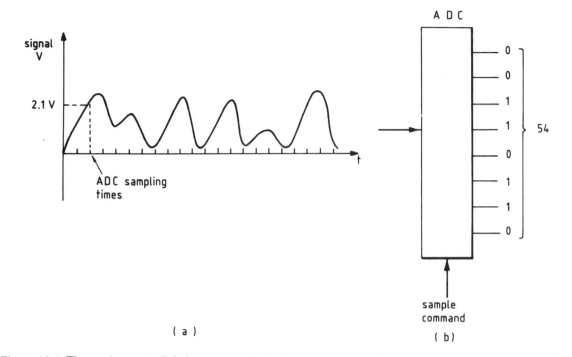

Figure 13.4 The analogue to digital converter (ADC). Input and sampling times (a) and ADC sample (b).

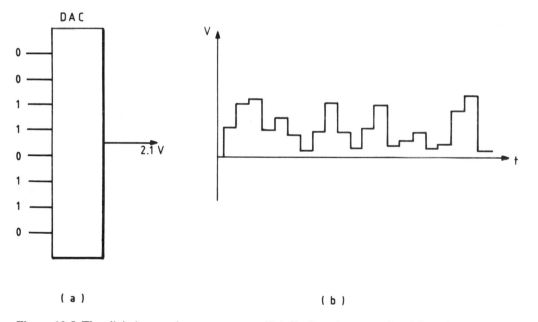

Figure 13.5 The digital to analogue converter (DAC). Sample conversion (a) and output (b).

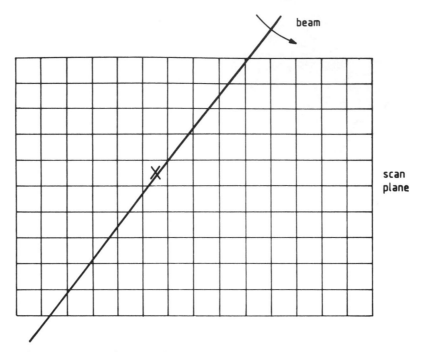

Figure 13.6 Division of the scan plane into small rectangular areas, each of which has a corresponding address in memory and rectangular display area (pixel) on the display monitor.

number representing its amplitude stored at the memory address representing that position and when the store contents are displayed on the video monitor a signal of intensity dependent on the stored echo amplitude will be displayed in the correct position.

13.8.2 Construction and Operation

A block diagram of the complete scan converter is shown in Figure 13.7. Echo signals are digitised by the ADC (some processing of the signal can take place at this stage) and the echoes from each beam position (scan line) are stored in a register prior to storage in the image memory. Information from the scanner on the beam and echo position is used to generate the correct address information for the memory. The memory is read a line at a time into a temporary video line register and following some further processing the information is converted into an analogue signal and sent to a video monitor. The timing of all these processes is under the control of a master timer.

13.8.3 Sampling Algorithms

The length of the beam within each pixel is not necessarily constant and the instrument will use a formula to decide the value which should be stored. For example, it may be the average of the echo amplitude along the line within the pixel. Alternatively, the value of the echo amplitude at a particular point on the beam may be shared amongst the nearest pixels on the basis of the distance of the centre of each pixel from the point, pixels with closer centres having a larger share.

13.8.4 Interpolation

Depending on the scan line density, some pixels will not be crossed by an ultrasound scan line

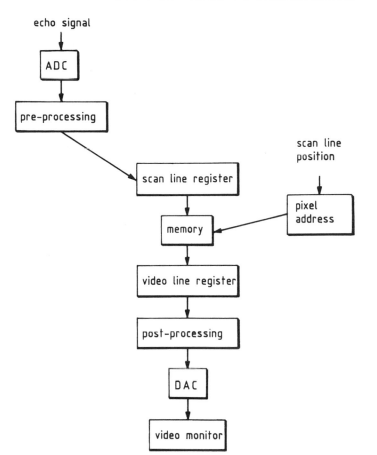

Figure 13.7 Scan converter block diagram.

(Figure 13.8), and it is usual to fill these pixels, to avoid spaces on the display, by a process of interpolation—calculating pixel contents on the basis of the echo amplitudes stored in nearby pixels. One method of interpolation, by no means the only one, is illustrated in Figure 13.8.

By interpolation, the calculated 'amplitude' for storage at address f is:

$$A_\mathrm{f} = \frac{1}{2} A_\mathrm{e} + \frac{1}{2} A_\mathrm{g} \qquad (13.1)$$

where A_e and A_g are the echo amplitudes stored at addresses 'e' and 'g' respectively.

Similarly, the 'amplitudes' stored at 'b' and 'c' are:

$$A_\mathrm{b} = \frac{2}{3} A_\mathrm{a} + \frac{1}{3} A_\mathrm{d}$$

and $\qquad (13.2)$

$$A_\mathrm{c} = \frac{1}{3} A_\mathrm{a} + \frac{2}{3} A_\mathrm{d}$$

13.8.5 Frame Freeze

It is possible using a scan converter to freeze an image, in which case the scan converter memory

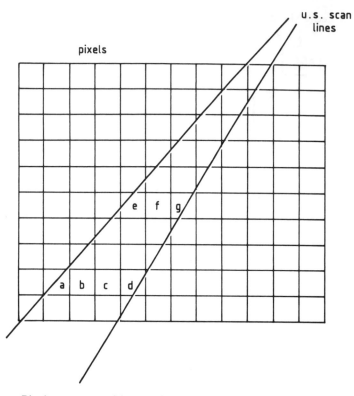

Figure 13.8 Interpolation. Pixels not crossed by an ultrasound scan line are 'filled' by interpolation using values in nearby pixels.

is continuously read out into the video monitor but no information is written from the ultrasound scanner.

13.9 DYNAMIC RANGE

The range of signal levels which can be stored is obviously limited by the number of bits in the scan converter memory. This is illustrated in Table 13.1.

13.10 PREPROCESSING

The range of echo amplitudes after time gain compensation is approximately 100:1 but in the interests of cost the scan converter memory may

Table 13.1 Maximum dynamic range for different numbers of bits.

Memory location size	Dynamic range
4 bits	15:1
6 bits	63:1
8 bits	255:1

have fewer bits than is required to cope with this. There are a number of ways of choosing the stored level from the echo signal range and this is known as preprocessing. Graphs representing the various methods of conversion from the digitised signal (usually 8 bits) to the stored levels (shown as 5 bits) are shown in Figure 13.9 and explained in Table 13.2.

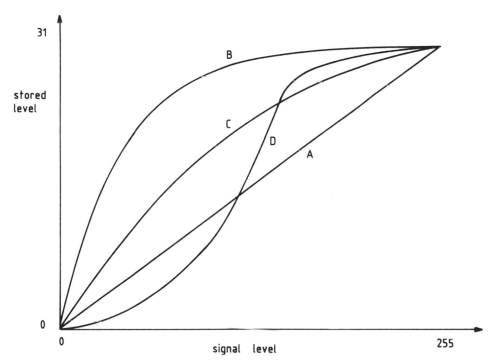

Figure 13.9 Preprocessing curves. Reproduced from McDicken, W.N. *Diagnostic Ultrasonics: Principles and Use of Instruments*, Churchill Livingstone, New York, 1981, with permission.

Table 13.2 Preprocessing curves.

Curve	Effect
A	Linear, even allocation of echo amplitudes.
B	Log compression, nearly all stored range allocated to low-level echoes, very little differentiation between high-level echoes.
C	Compression less severe, still emphasises low-level echoes.
D	Sigmoid, most of stored range for mid-range echoes.

13.11 FRAME AVERAGING

Frame averaging (correlation) is sometimes used to reduce the influence of background noise on picture quality. If successive frames (scans) are averaged, then noise will tend to cancel out whereas the image will be reinforced. Often several degrees of frame averaging are available on an instrument. In general, the new stored image level in any pixel store is a weighted average of the new image level and old values. For example, for 50% frame averaging:

Stored level = half old + half new

or for 75% frame averaging:

Stored level = three-quarters old + quarter new

The greater the weighting of the old stored value, the greater the number of frames contributing to each average and the more slowly the image is updated. A slow update rate will result in the image not following rapid changes, for example in imaging cardiac motion.

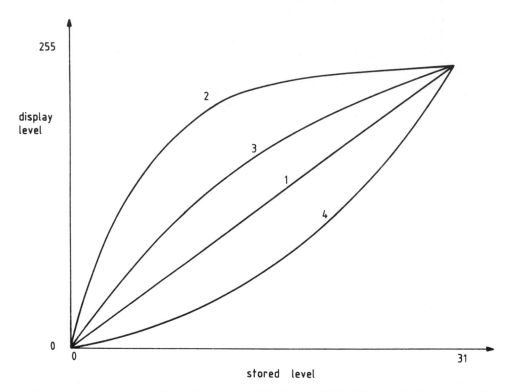

Figure 13.10 Post-processing curves. Reproduced from McDicken, W.N. *Diagnostic Ultrasonics: Principles and Use of Instruments*, Churchill Livingstone, New York, 1981, with permission.

13.12 POST-PROCESSING

The operator often has a choice of transfer function from stored to displayed value as shown in Figure 13.10. The transfer functions have the effects shown in Table 13.3.

Windowing will allow the operator to select only a small range of stored echo values to take up the whole of the display range.

Post-storage magnification (zoom) will allow a selected area of the stored image to occupy the whole of the display.

13.13 NUMBER OF PIXELS

The number of pixels used in the image will clearly have an effect on the image quality. An

Table 13.3 Postprocessing curves.

Curve	Effect
1	Linear, even allocation of echo amplitudes.
2	Compression of high-level echoes (high contrast).
3	Some compression of high-level echoes (medium contrast).
4	Compression of low-level echoes.

array of 512 by 512 will generally be unnoticeable but as the number reduces, the fact that the image is constructed of a number of squares or rectangles will be obvious and distracting. When the width of the pixels becomes comparable with the width of the ultrasound beam there will be degradation of resolution. The situation obviously becomes worse if post-storage magnification (zoom) is used, as a smaller number of stored pixels are used in the display.

13.14 NUMBER OF STORAGE LEVELS

The effect of the number of bits in the memory is shown in Figure 13.11. Obviously the lower the number of bits, the lower the number of digitised levels and the poorer the discrimination between echoes of different amplitude.

13.15 COMPUTATION ON STORED DATA

There is the potential for tissue characterisation by making use of characteristics of the stored B-scan image. For example, the computer can count the number of echoes having amplitudes in

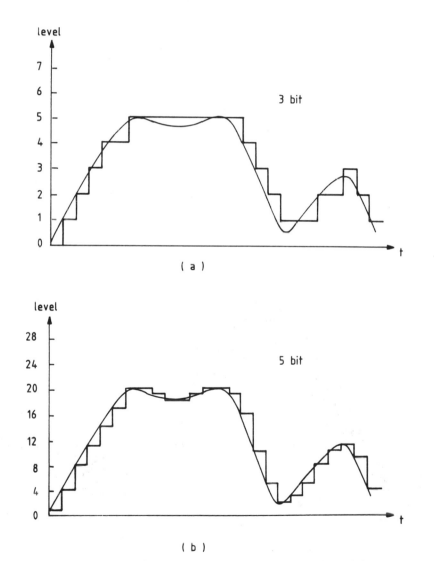

Figure 13.11 Signal digitisation using three (a) and five (b) bits.

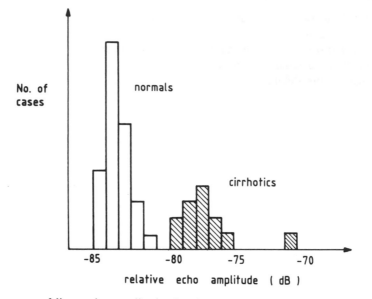

Figure 13.12 Case frequency of liver echo amplitude showing a separation between normal and cirrhotic liver. Reproduced, with permission, from Mountford, R.A. and Wells, P.N.T. (1972) Ultrasonic liver scanning: the A-scan in the normal and cirrhosis. *Physics in Medicine and Biology*, **17**, 261–269.

different amplitude ranges and plot these as a histogram. This has been shown to give different results for normal and cirrhotic livers, as shown in Figure 13.12. The attenuation in tissue may be calculated from the stored echo levels if the TGC and processing curves are taken into account. The number of echo maxima or minima within a small area, together with the contrast or

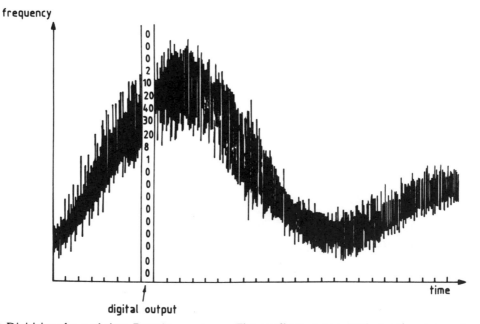

Figure 13.13 Digitising the real-time Doppler spectrum. The readings at one particular time interval are shown. The numbers represent the amplitude of the signal in each frequency interval.

range of echo levels, may be calculated. These figures will be dependent on tissue structure. The degree of change in the echo pattern from frame to frame under the influence of arterial pulsation can be measured and will depend, amongst other things, on the tissue compliance.

13.16 STORAGE OF, AND CALCULATIONS FROM, THE DOPPLER SPECTRUM

The real-time Doppler spectrum can be stored by digitising the amplitude of the signal at the different frequency levels at time intervals during the cardiac cycle, as shown in Figure 13.13. From these stored values can be calculated the maximum and mean frequency waveforms, spectral width and the various velocity waveform indices. The vessel angle and vessel width information may be used in conjunction with the stored spectrum data in order to calculate blood velocities and volume flow rates. If the information from a number of cardiac cycles is stored, then averages of the various measurements may be taken over a number of cardiac cycles.

CHAPTER 14

Image Artifacts

14.1 INTRODUCTION

A number of the properties of ultrasound and imaging instruments can lead to misleading effects in the ultrasound image. Ultrasound instruments generate images assuming that ultrasound travels in straight lines along beams having negligible thickness at a constant speed and that received echo amplitude is governed by the nature of the reflector in isolation. None of these assumptions is strictly valid. If the ultrasound beam is deviated by refraction and reflection and if the ultrasound velocity in parts of the tissue is different from that assumed by the instrument, images will be misplaced and/or distorted. Local variations in attenuation away from that assumed by the TGC setting will lead to spuriously high or low image intensities. On top of this, inappropriate control settings may lead to misleading images.

In this chapter, the various artifacts and their physical basis will be described.

14.2 MULTIPLE REFLECTIONS

14.2.1 In Tissue

A highly reflecting interface parallel to the transducer surface will give rise to multiple reflections—sometimes called reverberation—as shown in Figure 14.1. The ultrasound is reflected at both the interface and the probe surface, leading to multiple echoes displayed at integer multiples of the depth of the reflector. Each successive echo signal will be reduced in amplitude due to losses at each reflection and attenuation in the tissue. This multiple reflection can take place not only between an interface and probe surface but also between two highly reflecting interfaces.

Examples are reverberation between transducer and bowel gas, and transducer and anterior bladder wall.

The type of multiple reflection artifact seen on linear array B-scan images is shown in Figure 14.2a. If the gap between probe surface and reflector is small then the multiple echoes will often merge, leading to a wide bright band as shown in Figure 14.2b.

Figure 14.3 shows the reverberation echo intensities when reflection losses at the probe and interface are 50 and 70% respectively and there is 2-dB loss (63%) by attenuation between the probe and interface. In this case, five echoes will be displayed within a displayed dynamic range of 40 dB. With a 1% intensity reflection coefficient, which would be typical of a fat–muscle interface, the second echo is already 40 dB down on the first echo even before taking into account attenuation losses.

A second form of multiple reflection is shown in Figure 14.4 where the ultrasound pulse is reflected from one reflector (1) to a second (2) and then back to the probe. In addition to the signal directly from reflector 1, the instrument will see a second echo with a time of arrival indicating a slightly greater depth as shown. If reflector 1 is curved then the spurious image of reflector 2 will be distorted.

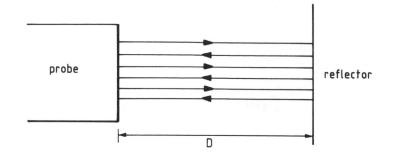

(a)

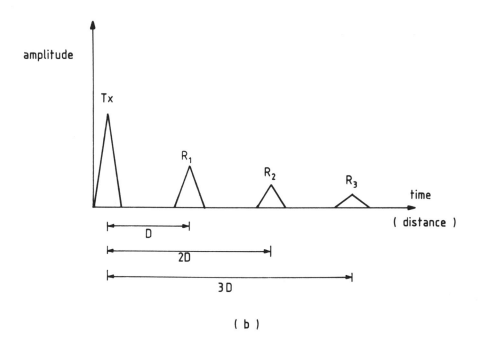

(b)

Figure 14.1 Multiple reflections. Probe/reflector geometry (a) and A-scan display (b).

Even when multiple reflection images cannot be clearly identified it is clear that this situation can occur at many places in the image, leading to multiple small spurious images, the net effect of which is to increase the background intensity of the image and reduce image contrast.

14.2.2 In the Probe

With reference to Figure 14.5a it is clear that multiple reflections can be formed between the transducer and the membrane in a mechanical real-time probe. This is particularly noticeable when the probe is held in the air as there is a large impedance mismatch at the membrane, giving rise to a high coefficient of reflection, but there is also an imperfect match between the probe and tissue when the transducer is applied to the skin surface and this mismatch can give rise to multiple reflections as shown. The problem can be alleviated by a careful choice of oil and membrane material having acoustic impedances close to that of tissue, or, as shown in Figure

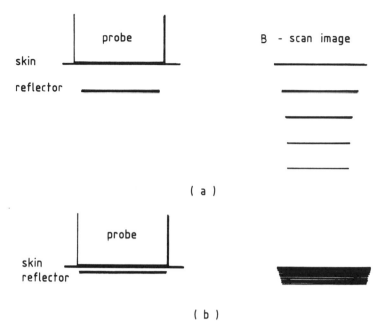

(a)

(b)

Figure 14.2 The B-scan image of multiple reflections with a large (a) and small (b) probe/reflector distance.

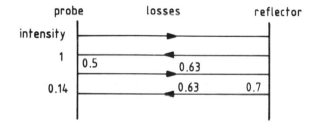

echo	intensity	(dB)
1	1	0
2	0.14	−8.5
3	0.02	−17
4	0.003	−25.5
5	0.0004	−34

Figure 14.3 Echo intensity reduction during multiple reflections. The intensity reflection coefficients at the probe and reflector are 0.5 and 0.7 respectively. The intensity is reduced by a factor of 0.63 through attenuation during each passage through tissue.

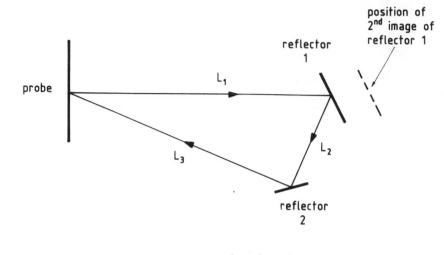

$$\text{Depth of } 2^{\text{nd}} \text{ image} = \frac{L_1 + L_2 + L_3}{2}$$

Figure 14.4 Multiple reflection via an off-axis reflector.

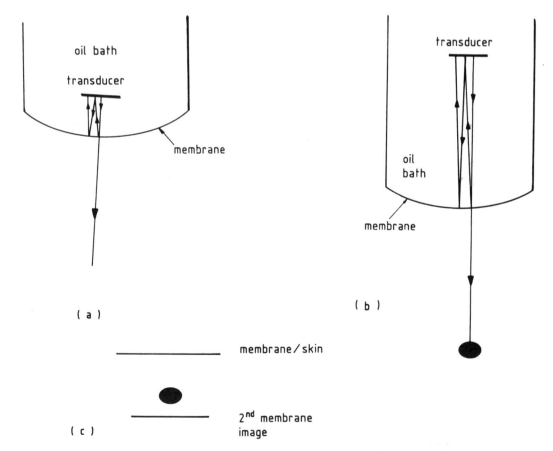

Figure 14.5 Multiple reflections within a mechanical real-time probe (a), increased transducer/membrane distance (b) and corresponding image (c).

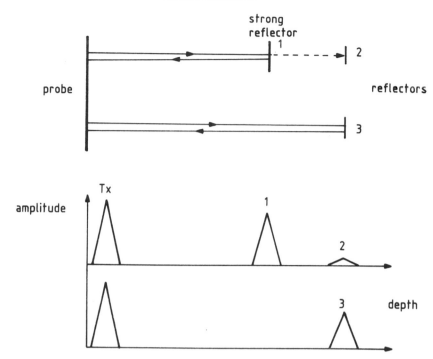

Figure 14.6 Shadowing behind a strong reflector. Probe/reflector geometry (a) and A-scan displays (b).

14.5b, by a large offset between the transducer and the membrane. If this distance is greater than the distance between the membrane and the deepest tissue to be imaged then the second membrane image will appear deeper than the bottom of the field of view and not interfere with the image (Figure 14.5c). The price to be paid, of course, is a very much more bulky probe.

14.3 SHADOWING

This artifact, illustrated in Figure 14.6, occurs whenever a strong reflector or absorber of ultrasound is present in the beam. Such a structure reduces the intensity of ultrasound travelling to and from reflectors and scatterers behind it and thereby reduces the amplitude of received echoes. The image of a strongly reflecting/attenuating

body in a uniform scattering region is shown in Figure 14.7.

Shadowing occurs behind bowel gas, bone, gall and kidney stones and highly attenuating tumours.

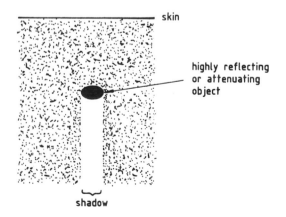

Figure 14.7 Shadowing by a highly reflecting or attenuating object in a uniform scattering region.

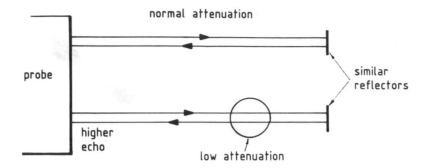

Figure 14.8 Low-attenuation enhancement. Probe/reflector geometry.

14.4 ENHANCEMENT (POST-CYSTIC)

This artifact is illustrated in Figure 14.8. It occurs when an ultrasound beam passes through a region of low attenuation, leading to reduced attenuation of the pulses transmitted to, and received from, reflectors on the far side of this region. The amplitudes of the echoes from behind such a region are clearly going to be higher than those from adjacent reflectors and scatterers. The image of a low-attenuation cyst in a uniform scattering region is shown in Figure 14.9.

14.5 BEAM WIDTH

The ultrasound scanner assigns a position on the screen to any echo received from a structure in

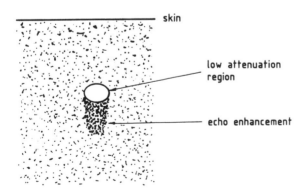

Figure 14.9 B-scan image of low-attenuation echo enhancement.

the beam according to the time of arrival of the echo and the position of the axis of the ultrasound beam. Images from structures within the beam but not on the axis are therefore misplaced. The effect of this is to elongate images by the width of the ultrasound beam. The process of generation of the image of a small reflector by a linear array is illustrated in Figure 14.10.

Since the beam width changes with depth the images of small objects will tend to be wide, close to and far away from the transducer, and narrow in the region of the focus.

14.6 SLICE WIDTH

The width of the beam perpendicular to the scan plane defines the slice width—shown for the case of a linear array in Figure 14.11. Reflectors within this slice will be imaged as if they were within the scan plane (the surface swept out by the beam axis) but with reduced amplitudes determined by the distance of the reflectors from the scan plane. The effect is to reduce the image contrast by the superposition of low-level echoes. This is particularly noticeable when imaging vessels in longitudinal section (as shown), when scatter from the lateral walls of the vessel will appear as low-intensity echoes within the vessel image.

14.7 TRANSMITTED PULSE LENGTH

There will be elongation of echoes along the beam as a result of the finite axial resolution

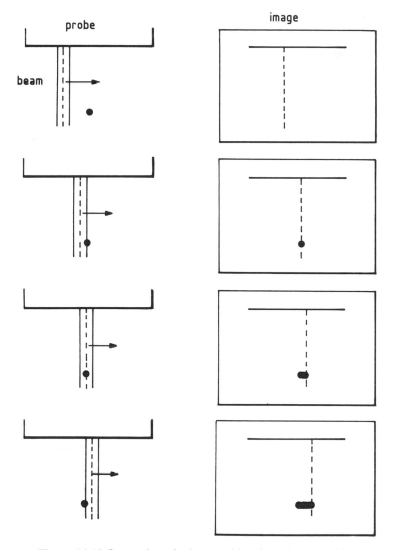

Figure 14.10 Image broadening resulting from beam width.

defined by the transmitted pulse length. Since axial resolution is far better than lateral resolution (defined by beam width) this effect is small.

14.8 REGISTRATION ERROR (VELOCITY DIFFERENCE)

This artifact is illustrated in Figure 14.12. If the characteristic velocity of the medium between two imaged interfaces is different from the calibration velocity (1540 m/s) then the spacing of the interface images will be in error since the instrument assigns depth simply on the basis of time of arrival of ultrasound pulses. If the velocity is higher, the echo from the distal interface will arrive after a shorter delay and the interface will be imaged closer than it should be. The converse will apply if the characteristic velocity is lower than the calibration velocity. An example is the displacement of the image of the retina towards the transducer as a result of the higher velocity of ultrasound in the lens of the eye than in the aqueous and vitreous humours.

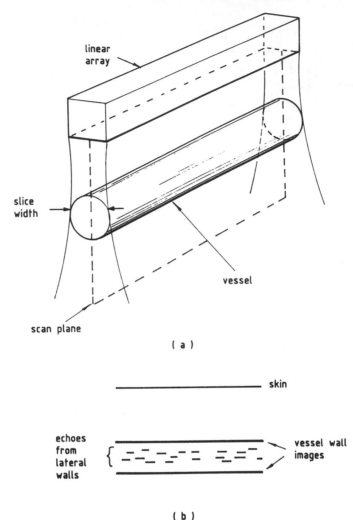

Figure 14.11 Spurious images resulting from finite slice width. Slice/vessel geometry (a) and vessel image showing spurious echoes from lateral walls (b).

14.9 REFRACTION

This artifact is again dependent on velocity differences and is illustrated in Figure 14.13. Refraction is the bending of the ultrasound beam when it passes through an interface between media of differing characteristic velocity. The degree of bending is governed by Snell's law (Section 3.3). Again the instrument will assign a position to the image of a reflector according to the time of arrival of the echo from that structure and the position of the beam. As can be seen in the figure, the image of a reflector can be displaced from its true position (clearly the distance of the image from the probe will also be displaced due to the effect illustrated in Figure 14.12). Refraction is important where there are significant deviations of velocity away from 1540 m/s. This can occur at the interface of fat with other soft tissues since fat has a characteristic

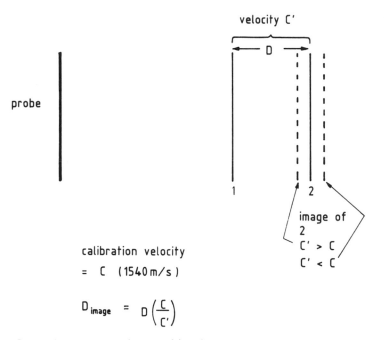

Figure 14.12 Error in reflector image separation resulting from a characteristic velocity between the reflectors being different from the calibration velocity of the instrument.

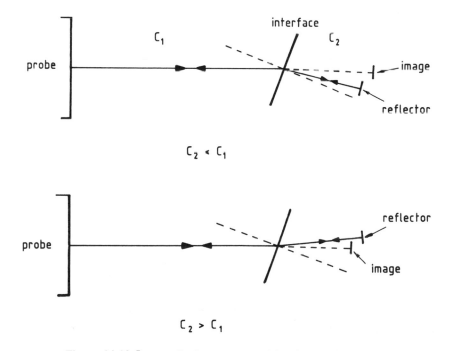

Figure 14.13 Image displacement resulting from refraction.

velocity of 1460 m/s, leading to refraction errors in breast imaging, for example. It will also occur in imaging the eye because of the relatively high velocity in the lens material (1620 m/s).

14.10 SIDE LOBES (see Section 4.2.3)

An instrument using a transducer with significant side lobes for imaging could be sensitive to echoes from structures well outside the main beam but such echoes would be assigned, by the instrument, to a position on the beam axis. The generation of such a spurious image is shown in Figure 14.14. A strong reflector at an angle to the main beam where the transducer has appreciable, although lower, sensitivity could generate an image on the screen of comparable intensity to the images of weak reflectors or scatterers in the main beam.

The position and size of the side lobes is determined by the shape and ratio of the size of the transducer to the wavelength. The side lobes can be reduced by apodisation in which it is arranged that the transducer pressure output (transmission) and sensitivity (reception) over the transducer surface are high at the centre and reduce towards the edges. This is clearly more easily implemented on annular arrays and linear array transducers than for single-element transducers.

14.11 GRATING LOBES (see Section 7.6)

These have the same form and lead to similar artifacts as side lobes but they are the property

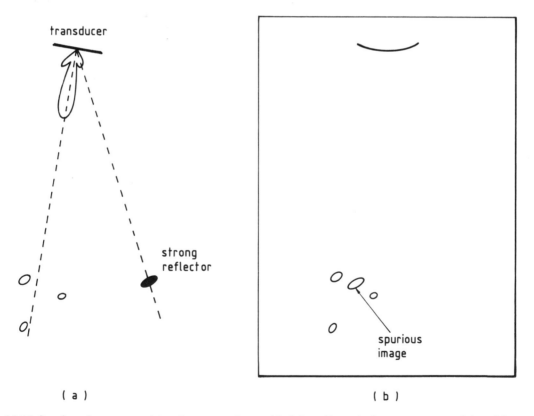

(a)   (b)

Figure 14.14 Spurious images resulting from transducer side lobes. Beam/reflector geometry (a) and image (b).

of the periodic nature of the construction of multiple-element transducers such as linear arrays and phased array transducers.

14.13 TGC MISUSE

The TGC control should be set to compensate for tissue attenuation and for beam sensitivity depth variation. Setting the control so that it over- or undercompensates will obviously give rise to misleading images.

14.14 SPECKLE

When imaging a region of tissue where scatterers are spaced at less than the axial resolving distance of the instrument, the echoes from individual scatterers interfere (see Section 5.7) and the peaks in the echo signal (determining the position of the image bright spots) are not in the same positions as would be determined by the individual echoes. Thus the image pattern is not the same as the scatterer pattern. This phenomenon is termed 'speckle'.

14.15 FRAME AVERAGING

As mentioned in Section 13.11, frame averaging should not be used when monitoring rapidly moving structures. For example, if frame averaging is used when imaging a heart valve, then weaker images of the valve in its position during previous frames will be shown together with the image of the valve in its current position.

14.16 M-MODE

Particular M-mode artifacts in cardiac studies are shadowing by rib or lung; reverberation between transducer and the posterior wall of the left ventricle, leading to a spurious trace beyond the heart echoes, with a range of movement twice that of the genuine heart wall echo; misleading valve movement traces arising from poor choice of orientation of the ultrasound beam, leading to insonation of different parts of the valve over its range of movement; and gaps in M-mode traces due to the movement of reflectors out of the beam at points during their movement.

CHAPTER 15

Performance Checks

15.1 INTRODUCTION

Many faults which develop on ultrasound scanners are obvious to the user. However, there are some faults, particularly gradual changes in performance, which may not be detected except by routine performance checks.

We will deal, in this chapter, specifically with checks on imaging instruments. Methods of monitoring Doppler and M-mode performance have been described elsewhere. It should also be noted that as a part of, or separately from, the performance checks, an electrical safety check should be carried out on ultrasound instruments to ensure that potentially dangerous electrical faults have not developed. This is particularly important with machines using intracavity and intraoperative probes where the potential for lethal shock is much higher if the electrical insulation of the probe has been compromised.

Routine performance checks can be carried out to measure sensitivity, dynamic range, dead zone, registration, resolution, geometric distortion on displays and hard copy devices, and caliper accuracy.

Sensitivity and dynamic range can be reduced by damage to the transducer, an increase in noise level in the receiver circuits, a reduction in transmitter output power and a reduction in gain in receiver amplifiers.

The dead zone, as we have seen previously, is caused by reverberation within the probe and can be increased by probe damage or faults in the electrical matching and damping circuits connected to the transducer.

Registration (the ability of the instrument to place the image of a tissue structure in the right place on the screen) is compromised by mechanical faults in the scanning arms of static B-scanners, changes in the velocity calibration and changes in the circuits connected with image positioning.

Resolution can be affected by damage to the transducers (alterations to the transducer geometry will alter the beam shape) and faults in the electronic focussing circuits.

Geometric distortion on the display and hard copy units can be caused by faults in the raster scanning circuits in the video monitors.

Caliper calibration can be affected by changes in the velocity calibration and faults in marker positioning and distance calculation circuits.

15.2 CONTROL SETTINGS

The importance of control settings in the use of test objects cannot be overemphasised. During any test all controls affecting the image quality, other than those altered as part of the test, should be set to standard settings, by reference to the image or from the setting of the relevant control. Only in this way can reproducible results be achieved and changes in performance detected. Specifically, the controls which require standard settings are brightness, contrast, TGC, transmitter power, receiver gain, reject or dynamic range and pre- and post-processing controls.

15.3 PERSPEX BLOCK TEST OBJECT

The simplest test object is a perspex block a few centimetres thick as shown in Figure 15.1a. Multiple reflections are observed as shown and the device may be used as a rough monitor of sensitivity by noting the setting of either the transmitter output or the receiver gain control required to reduce a particular echo image just to the point of extinction. The dynamic range may be monitored by noting the range over which the relevant control has to be moved to vary the displayed echo intensity from the point at which it just disappears to a peak white display. The velocity calibration of the display instrument may be checked by noting the separation of the echoes on the screen, bearing in mind that the higher velocity (2680 m/s) in perspex means that 1.74 cm of perspex is equivalent to 1 cm of tissue (1540 m/s). Similarly, the velocity calibration of the calipers may be checked by setting the caliper markers on the displayed echoes. In use, a small amount of oil or coupling jelly is used on the surface of the perspex block and the transducer probe is rocked backwards and forwards until the displayed echoes are at a maximum.

15.4 STANDARD VELOCITY FLUID BATH

Similar measurements can be made using a reflector in a bath of fluid with an ultrasound velocity of 1540 m/s (e.g. 10% ethyl alcohol in degassed water at 20°C). Since temperature variations of the fluid will alter the ultrasound velocity, corrections may have to be made if the temperature of the bath is significantly different from 20°C.

15.5 THE AIUM TEST RIG

15.5.1 Construction

In order to carry out more accurate checks of a wide range of performance characteristics, a more complex test object is required. A suitable object consists of a series of stainless steel wires or

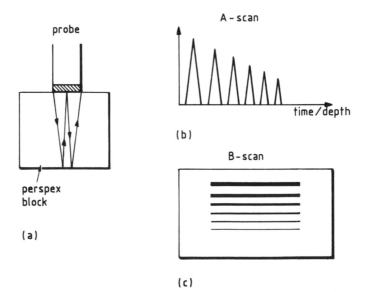

Figure 15.1 Performance checks using a perspex block. Probe/block geometry (a), A-scan display (b) and B-scan display (c).

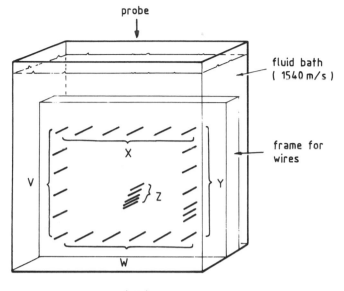

probe

fluid bath
(1540 m/s)

frame for
wires

(a)

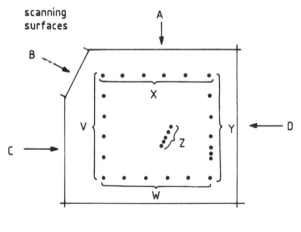

scanning
surfaces

(b)

Figure 15.2 AIUM test objects. Open top (a) and enclosed (b). Reproduced, with permission, from Goldstein, A. (1980) *Quality Assurance in Diagnostic Ultrasound. A Quality Assurance Manual for the Clinical User.* © 1980 by American Institute of Ultrasound in Medicine.

nylon threads stretched over a frame within a bath of 1540 m/s characteristic velocity fluid. The American Institute of Ultrasound in Medicine (AIUM) test rig is shown in Figure 15.2. There are two forms. In the first (Figure 15.2a) the wire frame is inserted into a bath containing the standard velocity fluid and measurements are carried out with the transducer face immersed in the fluid. The second version (Figure 15.2b) is enclosed and has three flexible plastic sonic windows to which the probe under test is applied using a coupling medium.

15.5.2 Sensitivity and Dynamic Range

Sensitivity and dynamic range may be monitored as with the perspex block—selecting the echo from a mid-range wire.

15.5.3 Dead Zone

The superficial X wires gradually increase in depth and are used for dead zone measurement. The dead zone thickness is given by the depth of the first wire visible (Figure 15.3).

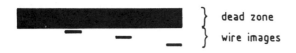

Figure 15.3 B-scan image of X wires during dead zone measurement.

15.5.4 Caliper Accuracy

Vertical caliper accuracy is checked by lining up the caliper markers on echoes from the V or Y wires and comparing the displayed reading with the known separation of these wires. The horizon-tal caliper accuracy may be checked by setting the caliper markers on echoes from the W wires. The caliper accuracy should be 2% or better in 10 cm or limited only by the number of digits displayed by the caliper.

There is a potential problem when measuring horizontal caliper accuracy using mechanical sector scanners on enclosed test objects. Coupling jelly may have a significantly different characteristic velocity from the standard and when used to provide coupling into a test object by using a wedge of jelly, as illustrated in Figure 15.4, there may be significant errors due to refraction at the jelly–test object window surface. This can be eliminated by either using an open-top test object with mechanical sector scanners or filling the tray surrounding the test object window with a standard velocity fluid for coupling purposes.

15.5.5 Axial Resolution

Axial resolution is measured using the Z wires. These wires have a gradually decreasing separation. They are set at a slight angle to the perpendicular to avoid shadowing. The resolution is noted as the separation of the closest pair of wires whose images can be separated on the

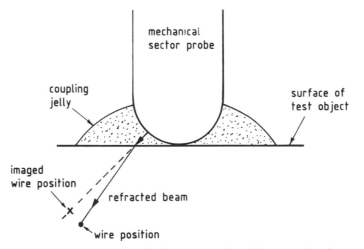

Figure 15.4 Refraction error when using mechanical sector probe with an enclosed test object. Adapted, with permission, from Price, R. (1986) Geometric distortion in quality control images from sector scanners. In: J.A. Evans (ed.) *Physics in Medical Ultrasound*, Report No. 47, Institute of Physical Sciences in Medicine.

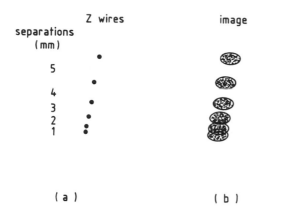

Figure 15.5 Axial resolution measurement using Z wires. Wire geometry (a), and image (b).

screen (Figure 15.5). The axial resolution should normally be less than or equal to three wavelengths at the frequency of the transducer under test.

15.5.6 Lateral Resolution

Lateral resolution can be measured in two ways. As shown in Figure 15.6a, the width of the image of the V wires is an indication of beam width and therefore lateral resolution at different depths. Alternatively, as shown in Figure 15.6b, the Y wires may be scanned by rotating the wire frame in the open-top test object, or by scanning from the side in the enclosed test object, and noting

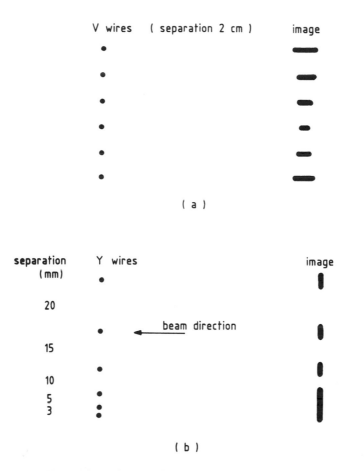

Figure 15.6 Beam width and lateral resolution measurement using V wires (a) and Y wires (b).

the separation of the closest pair of resolvable wire images.

To ensure comparability and repeatability of results when making resolution measurements, the displayed echo level of the wires should be similar for all measurements and the gain controls should be set to ensure this.

15.5.7 Registration

The registration of a static B-scanner may be tested as shown in Figure 15.7a by scanning the wires from the two extreme edges of the tank of the open-top test object, in which case correct registration is demonstrated if the two echo lines for each wire bisect one another, as shown. A somewhat more rigorous check may be carried out using the enclosed test object by (Figure 15.7b) scanning the enclosed wires from three directions, in which case the three scan lines should all bisect each other, meeting at a point. The depth registration on both static B-scan and real-time scanners can be checked by noting the position of the images of the V wires.

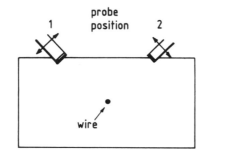

(a)

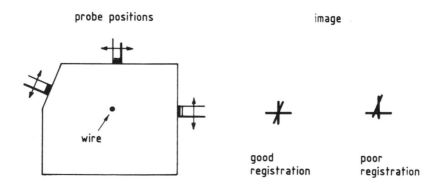

(b)

Figure 15.7 Static B-scan registration check using an open-top (a) and enclosed (b) test object.

15.6 THE CARDIFF RESOLUTION TEST RIG

15.6.1 Introduction

One of the drawbacks of the test object described is that the medium is non-attenuating so that the instrument is not being tested under realistic conditions. The more advanced enclosed test objects contain a stable gel with a characteristic velocity of 1540 m/s, loaded with material to give attenuation with a typical frequency dependence (usually of the order of 1 dB cm^{-1} MHz^{-1}) and containing small scattering particles to give a scatter background image.

15.6.2 Construction

The wire arrangements for one such device, the Cardiff resolution test object, is shown in Figure 15.8.

15.6.3 Registration, Dead Zone and Caliper Accuracy

Registration, dead zone and caliper accuracy are tested in a fashion similar to that described for the AIUM test rig. The area calculation capability of the instrument may be checked using the calipers and tracing out a shape defined by selected A and B wires.

15.6.4 Penetration

Sensitivity is measured by means of a measurement of penetration. Imaging the B wires from surface 1, the transmitter output is set to a maximum and the receiver gain and TGC controls adjusted to give a uniform background scatter image to as great a depth as possible. The depth, as indicated by the B wires or by a caliper measurement, at which only 30% of each small area of the screen is occupied by background scatter image (the rest of the area being dark) is taken as the low-contrast penetration. A measurement of high-contrast penetration is the depth of the last B wire which can be identified (Figure 15.9).

15.6.5 Resolution

The setting-up procedure for resolution measurements using this test object is as follows.

The swept gain, transmitter output and receiver gain controls are set as for the penetration measurement and then the transmitter output (and if necessary the receiver gain) is reduced until 70% of each small area of the background image is dark. The axial resolution at a range of depths is measured using the D wires, noting the separation of the closest pair of separable wire images as in the AIUM test rig axial resolution test. The lateral resolution can again be measured by noting the widths of the B-wire images, or, alternatively, by noting the separation of the closest pair of resolvable E-wire images, at a range of different depths (Figure 15.10).

15.6.6 Slice Thickness

Slice thickness at different depths can be measured using the F wires, which run in a direction parallel to the scanning plane. The scanning arrangement is shown in Figure 15.11. For each group of F wires, the probe is rocked slightly and the minimum number of imaged wires noted. The estimate of the slice thickness is given by the number of wires imaged and their horizontal separation.

15.7 OTHER TEST OBJECTS

Other test objects, which can also be used as phantoms for demonstration and teaching purposes, have been constructed with regions of low scatter and low attenuation, simulating cysts, and higher attenuation and scatter, simulating metastases, set in standard scatter and attenuation

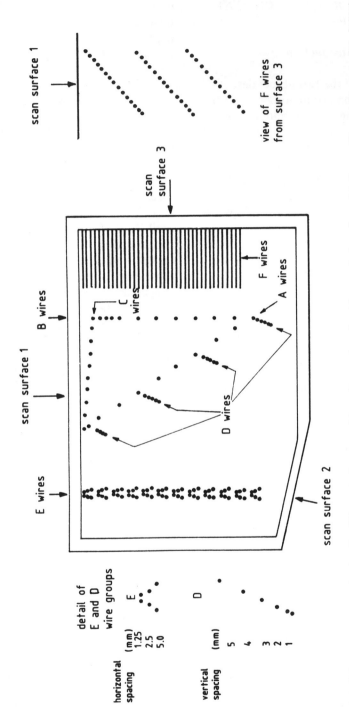
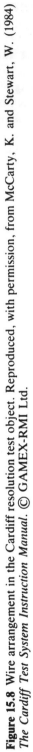

Figure 15.8 Wire arrangement in the Cardiff resolution test object. Reproduced, with permission, from McCarty, K. and Stewart, W. (1984) *The Cardiff Test System Instruction Manual.* © GAMEX-RMI Ltd.

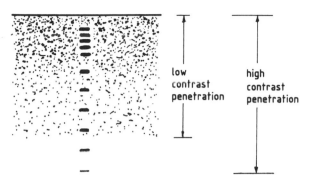

Figure 15.9 Measurement of low-contrast and high-contrast penetration using the Cardiff test object.

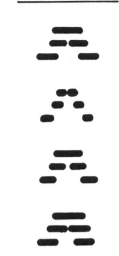

Figure 15.10 Lateral resolution measurement using the E wires in the Cardiff test object.

material. The performance of instruments can be qualitatively assessed by checking that cysts appear clear and that the lateral walls are clearly defined and that there is post-cystic enhancement. High-scatter regions should be clearly identified together with shadowing. Step wedges of higher attenuating and scattering material may be used for greyscale range evaluation.

15.8 GEOMETRIC DISTORTION

Geometric distortion on displays and hard copy units can be checked by scanning a rectangular

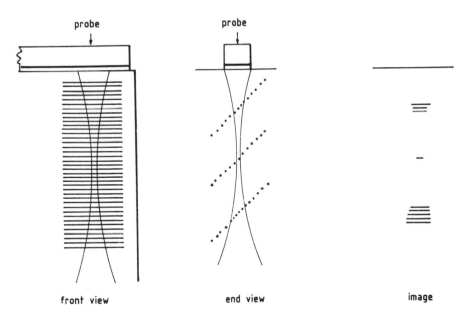

Figure 15.11 Slice width measurement using the F wires in the Cardiff test object. Reproduced, with permission, from McCarty, K. and Stewart, W. (1984) *The Cardiff Test System Instruction Manual.* © GAMEX-RMI Ltd.

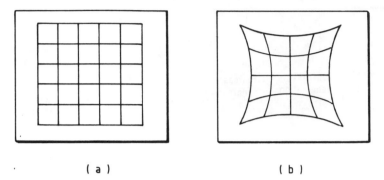

(a)   (b)

Figure 15.12 Display distortion using a grid test pattern showing an example of a correct display (a) and pin cushion distortion (b).

grid of wires and checking the spacing of the wires at all points on the screen and hard copy. A simpler method is to check these devices separately from the ultrasound scanner using a video test pattern generator, which can generate a greyscale wedge for dynamic range assessment and a square pattern for distortion measurement (Figure 15.12).

15.9 DOCUMENTATION

As with all routine checks on instrument performance, clear documentation and, where possible, hard copy of the images obtained will ease the identification of faults.

CHAPTER 16

Bioeffects, Dosimetry and Safety

16.1 INTRODUCTION

We have, in previous chapters, considered the effects of different tissues on ultrasound. There is another aspect to the interaction of ultrasound and tissues and that is the effect that the ultrasound has on the tissues. Tissues can be altered or damaged by ultrasound of sufficiently high intensity by the physical damage mechanisms listed below:

Heating
Radiation force
Streaming
Stable cavitation
Transient (collapse) cavitation
Standing wave effects
Non-linear effects
Direct effects

From investigations of these physical mechanisms and their biological effects, we need to determine safe levels of ultrasound for diagnostic purposes and we need reliable methods of measuring the output of ultrasound instruments in order to ensure that these levels are not exceeded.

16.2 PHYSICAL DAMAGE MECHANISMS

16.2.1 Heating

Ultrasound is attenuated during its passage through tissue, due to scatter and absorption. The major component of attenuation in all tissues is absorption by relaxation and visco-elastic effects leading to heating of the tissue.

It is found (see Appendix F) that the temperature of an insonated (irradiated with ultrasound) volume of tissue initially increases linearly with time after the ultrasound is switched on. The rate of temperature increase is proportional to the ultrasound intensity and the absorption coefficient of the tissue, and inversely proportional to its heat capacity and density. The linear rise in temperature does not continue, however. As the temperature of the tissue volume rises, it loses heat by conduction through the surrounding tissue, through convective cooling by flowing blood and, if close to the skin surface, by radiation from the skin. If we measure the temperature rise during insonation then we get graphs similar to those shown in Figure 16.1. The temperature will start to rise at a rate indicated by the dashed lines and will reach an equilibrium temperature which increases with intensity and absorption coefficient and decreases with the degree of cooling (Figure 16.2).

For the same intensity (not power) a small insonated region of tissue (e.g. within a focussed ultrasound beam) will have a lower equilibrium temperature at the centre than will a larger region (e.g. from an unfocussed beam). This is illustrated in Figure 16.3. This is because the capacity to store heat is proportional to the volume of the tissue and therefore increases as the cube of the linear dimensions of the tissue volume, whereas the ability to lose heat is related to the surface area, which increases only as the square of the linear dimensions of the tissue volume.

The heating effect is also affected by the duty cycle of the ultrasound beam. If the ultrasound is not on continuously but is periodically switched

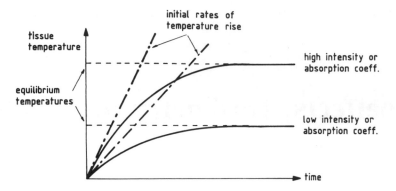

Figure 16.1 Temperature rise in tissue during insonation.

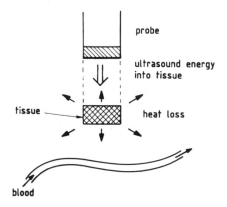

Figure 16.2 Ultrasound energy absorption in, and heat loss from, insonated tissue.

on and off (a typical regime is 4 ms on and 4 ms off) then the duty cycle is the percentage of the total time that the ultrasound is switched on. Since cooling can take place during the off periods, it is to be expected that the duty cycle of the ultrasound will influence any thermal effects.

A particularly rapid loss of energy with distance leading to high local heating is thought to arise from a phenomenon called mode conversion. When ultrasound passes from soft tissue into bone, some of the ultrasound energy goes into vibrating the bone in a transverse fashion (shear wave) as shown in Figure 16.4. Part of the shear wave is emitted into the soft tissue and since soft

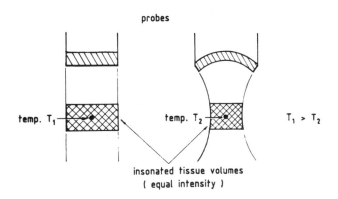

Figure 16.3 The dependence of equilibrium temperature on the volume of the insonated tissue.

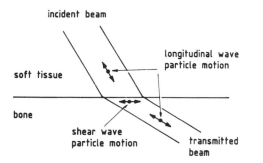

Figure 16.4 Mode conversion at a soft tissue–bone interface.

tissue cannot easily support a shear wave it is very strongly attenuated. This leads to a power loss in a very thin layer of tissue close to the bone surface, leading to a high temperature.

16.2.2 Radiation Force

This is the force on any absorbing or reflecting object in an ultrasound beam.

For a perfect reflector, perpendicular to the beam, the force is:

$$F_r = \frac{2IA}{c} \quad \text{N} \qquad (16.1)$$

and for a perfect absorber:

$$F_a = \frac{IA}{c} \quad \text{N} \qquad (16.2)$$

where A is the area of the reflector or absorber intercepted by the beam.

This effect can be expressed in terms of radiation pressure (force per unit area). Then for a perfect reflector:

$$P_r = F_r/A = \frac{2I}{c} \quad \text{N/m}^2 \text{ or Pa} \qquad (16.3)$$

and for a perfect absorber:

$$P_a = \frac{I}{c} \quad \text{Pa} \qquad (16.4)$$

Or, since $IA = W$ (power):

$$F_r = \frac{2W}{c} \quad \text{N} \qquad (16.5)$$

$$F_a = \frac{W}{c} \quad \text{N} \qquad (16.6)$$

For example, the force on a perfect reflector in water at 20°C ($c = 1480$ m/s) is equivalent to 138 mg weight/W.

16.2.3 Streaming

This is another manifestation of radiation force. The ultrasound absorbed in a fluid gives rise to a force acting on the fluid which causes it to move in the direction of the ultrasound beam and this is known as streaming. It can be demonstrated by observing the motion of small particles or dye streams within an insonated fluid. The path of fluid motion, due to streaming, in front of an ultrasound transducer within a closed vessel, is shown in Figure 16.5. There is the potential for damage due to streaming as a result of the translational force on a fluid element, a

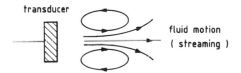

Figure 16.5 Streaming in the ultrasound field in an enclosed vessel.

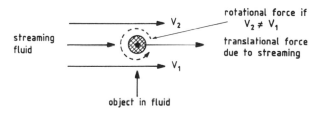

Figure 16.6 Translational force due to viscous drag, and torque due to velocity shear, on an object in an insonated fluid.

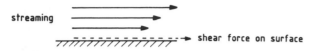

Figure 16.7 Surface shear force resulting from streaming.

torque or rotational force due to a velocity gradient or difference in velocity across the element (Figure 16.6) and a sheer force on surfaces within the moving fluid (Figure 16.7).

16.2.4 Cavitation

This is the growth and oscillation of bubbles within an ultrasound field (Figure 16.8). There are two types—stable cavitation and transient or collapse cavitation.

16.2.4.1 Stable Cavitation

Small bubbles grow by a process called rectified diffusion whereby vapour diffuses into a bubble during rarefaction and out during compression. Since the surface area of the bubble is larger

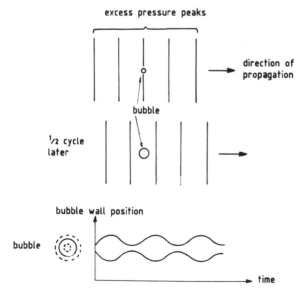

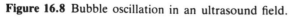

Figure 16.8 Bubble oscillation in an ultrasound field.

during the rarefaction phase of the cycle, there is a net inflow of vapour into the bubble, leading to an increase in size over several cycles of the ultrasound field. When the bubbles reach a certain size (proportional to wavelength), they resonate with the ultrasound, leading to a large increase in oscillation amplitude.

Approximately 1000 cycles are required for a bubble to grow to resonance at 1 MHz.

The motion of the bubble wall during oscillation causes rapid movement of the fluid in the region of the bubble. This is known as microstreaming and is thought to be a major cause of damage associated with stable cavitation.

16.2.4.2 Transient or Collapse Cavitation

At higher excess pressures bubble growth and violent collapse can take place within one or two cycles. The violent collapse of the bubble creates shock waves and very high temperatures, light emission and the formation of free radicals. The bubble collapse creates small bubble fragments as shown in Figure 16.9 which act as new nuclei (starting bubbles) for further cavitation.

Damage is caused by the high temperatures and tissue disruption by the shock waves. The free radicals (extremely reactive chemical species) cause damage by reacting with biochemicals within the tissue.

16.2.4.3 Detection of Cavitation

Cavitation can be detected by the emission from the insonated fluid of signals at half the frequency (a subharmonic) of the incident ultrasound, harmonics of the ultrasound frequency and 'white' noise (a signal consisting of a wide range of frequencies), the emission of light

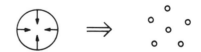

Figure 16.9 Bubble collapse and break-up during transient cavitation.

(sonoluminescence) and the effect of free radicals (sonochemistry)—for example, the release of free iodine from potassium iodide due to the action of the .OH radical formed from the splitting of water molecules. Large cavitation bubbles can be detected optically in clear media and an 8-MHz ultrasound scanner has been used to image bubbles *in vivo*.

16.2.4.4 Cavitation Threshold

The excess pressure of the ultrasound field must exceed a certain threshold level for cavitation to take place and this is known as the cavitation threshold.

The threshold depends on the presence of bubbles within the insonated media. Figure 16.10 shows the intensity of cavitation as detected by subharmonic emission in degassed and non-degassed water, showing a very much lower threshold in the water having dissolved air.

The threshold increases as the ambient pressure increases. This can be used as a test that a particular effect is due to cavitation if the effect disappears or reduces when the ambient pressure is increased.

The threshold also increases with temperature and with the viscosity of the cavitating liquid. This means that it should be more difficult to cause cavitation in biological fluids than in water.

It has also been noted that the cavitation threshold has a strong dependence on pulse duration, it being more difficult to cause cavitation with short pulses. Presumably, this is because a number of cycles are required for bubble growth. It should be noted, however, that the cavitation level as measured by iodine release from potassium iodide increases to a peak at certain pulse lengths, depending on the ultrasound frequency, before reducing again. It may be that the time constants involved in different chemical reactions initiated by free radical action may result in

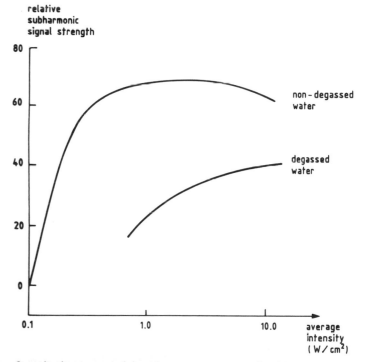

Figure 16.10 Degree of cavitation assessed by the measurement of subharmonic signal strength, against the intensity of ultrasound for degassed and non-degassed water. Adapted, with permission, from Hill, C.R. (1972) Ultrasonic exposure thresholds for changes in cells and tissues. *Journal of the Acoustical Society of America*, **52**, 667–672.

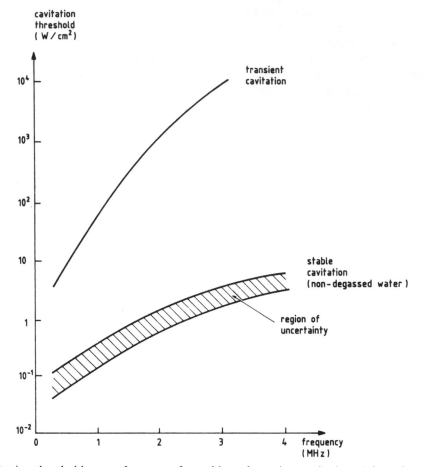

Figure 16.11 Cavitation threshold versus frequency for stable and transient cavitation. Adapted, with permission, from Hill, C.R. (1972) Ultrasonic exposure thresholds for changes in cells and tissues. *Journal of the Acoustical Society of America*, **52**, 667–672.

different optimum pulse lengths.

The cavitation threshold increases with frequency. The variation with frequency for stable and transient cavitation in air-equilibrated water is shown in Figure 16.11.

on compressible small structures in a standing wave field, moving them towards the pressure nodes (points of minimum excess pressure). This force will be expected to act on tissues within a standing wave field.

16.2.5 Standing Wave Effects

The reflection of ultrasound from a surface spaced an integer number of half-wavelengths from the transducer leads to a standing wave pattern as illustrated in Figure 16.12 as a result of constructive interference between the incident and reflected wave. It is found that there is a force

16.2.6 Non-Linear Effects

The assumption made up to now in our discussion of ultrasound fields is that there is a linear relationship between excess pressure and local density variations, due to the passage of the wave. At high excess pressures, as often found in the short pulses in imaging systems at high

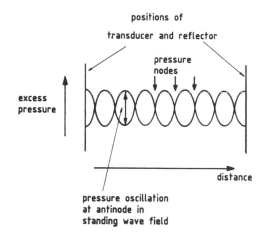

Figure 16.12 The pressure standing wave between the transducer and reflector separated by an integer number of half-wavelengths.

transmitted output levels, this linear relationship no longer holds. One of the effects of non-linearity is that the speed of propagation of positive excess pressure half-cycles is greater than the speed of propagation of the negative half-

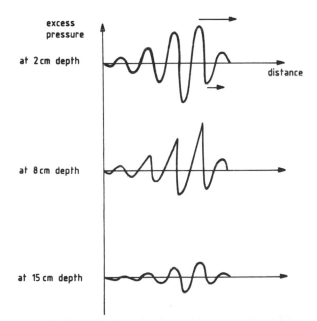

Figure 16.13 The development of pulse waveform distortion as a result of non-linear propagation and its reduction resulting from frequency-dependent attenuation.

cycles, as illustrated in Figure 6.13. This means that the positive pressure half-cycle will tend to catch up with the negative half-cycle, creating a very rapid change of pressure with distance, called a shock wave. This shock wave can form in approximately 7–10 cm in low-attenuation media. This distorted wave contains a higher proportion of high-frequency components than the initial wave and these are selectively attenuated by the frequency-dependent attenuation of tissue, leading to a low-amplitude pulse without a shock wave at a greater depth.

There is the potential for tissue damage due to the rapid change of pressure during the shock wave passage, an increased thermal effect due to the increased attenuation of the high-frequency components of the shock wave and also a net force acting parallel to the direction of travel of the pulse due to the difference in pressure gradients at the increasing and decreasing parts of the excess pressure pulse. This force is called the Oseen force.

16.2.7 Stokes Force

Small objects in an insonated medium tend to move in an oscillatory fashion with the particles in the medium as a result of viscous coupling (friction between the medium and the object). Because viscosity changes with temperature, and there are small oscillatory changes in temperature in sympathy with the pressure wave in the medium, the viscous force on any object within the medium is different during rarefaction and compression, leading to a net force on the object, parallel to the direction of propagation of the wave.

16.2.8 Bernoulli Force

Whenever moving fluids pass through a constriction—for example streaming fluid passing between two structures as shown in Figure 16.14—there is a force acting on the walls of the constriction towards the centre of the fluid stream.

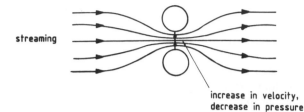

streaming

increase in velocity,
decrease in pressure

Figure 16.14 The Bernoulli forces on surfaces forming a constriction within a streaming fluid.

This results from the conservation of energy within the fluid. The fluid has potential energy related to its pressure and kinetic energy related to its velocity and the sum of these two energies is constant within each small volume of fluid. Since the velocity of the fluid increases as it passes through a constriction, the kinetic energy increases and therefore the potential energy (and therefore the pressure within the fluid) must decrease to maintain the total energy at a constant value. The sides of the constriction therefore try to move into the low-pressure region, giving rise to the force indicated.

16.3 BIOEFFECTS

16.3.1 Introduction

The relative importance of these different physical damage mechanisms in their biological effects is often unclear. It is, therefore, more convenient to categorise the biological effects according to the type of biological structure under investigation. The categories investigated are:

(1) Molecules/macromolecules in solution (DNA, proteins).
(2) Cells in suspension (HELA cells, human fibroblasts).
(3) Tissues *in vitro* and *in vivo* (excised liver, muscle).
(4) Whole body (fetal mice/rats *in utero*, epidemiology).

There is now a huge literature on bioeffects but a problem for anyone trying to draw conclusions is that many effects reported cannot be independently repeated. Often, reported effects do not result from action of the ultrasound but from some other aspect of the experiment. There is also a problem of a large number of variables which makes comparison of experiments difficult. These variables include frequency, intensity, volume insonated, whether fluids and suspensions are stirred or unstirred, the time of insonation, duty cycle of the radiation, ambient temperature and pressure and the type of molecule or tissue. There can be under- or overestimation of intensity due to inadvertent focussing or defocussing of the ultrasound beam passing across curved interfaces between media of different characteristic velocity or reflection at curved surfaces, and unintended standing waves in the tissue or suspension sample holder.

Experiments to determine the biological effect of a physical or chemical mechanism have a certain recognised structure. Firstly, since biological materials have a variable response to any intervention, it is necessary to repeat experiments on a number of samples and to measure an average effect. Secondly, to eliminate aspects of the experiment other than the intervention (e.g. temperature, container shape, pressure), samples are divided into two groups called the exposed and the control groups and the treatment of the two groups is the same in all respects except that the exposed group will suffer the intervention and the control group will not. For example, in testing the effect of ultrasound on a suspension of cells in a container, the control samples will be placed in and taken out of the container and treated in exactly the same way as the exposed group, except that the ultrasound will not be turned on. An effect of exposure can be said to have been detected when there is a difference between an observed effect in the exposed and control groups of samples and statistical tests have indicated that this difference cannot be attributable to mere chance. This latter requirement, in general, means that large numbers of samples are required for the detection of small effects, whereas large effects can be detected with a smaller number of samples. There is even a problem in the example outlined in that we must make sure that heat from the transducer, when the ultrasound is switched on, does not reach the sample, otherwise the temperature in the control and exposed groups will be different.

Our particular interest, of course, in carrying out experiments on the biological effect is to find out the effect on humans and thereby lies another problem in that we have to extrapolate from effects observed *in vitro* and on isolated cells and tissues in animals and plants to humans. In fact, tissues appear to show different sensitivity from isolated cells as a result of their physical structure, and different animals and plant cells show different sensitivity to ultrasound. It is recognised that this may often be due not only to different initial damage sensitivity but also to the differing efficiency of damage repair mechanisms within the tissue.

16.3.2 Molecules in Solution

Enzyme and DNA molecules in solution can be disrupted by ultrasound, but only at cavitation levels. As we have seen, the cavitation threshold is very much lower in the presence of dissolved air and small bubbles and this is reflected in thresholds for macromolecule disruption. Genetic damage from this source *in vivo* is likely to require very much higher ultrasound intensities since the cavitation thresholds will be higher in organised tissues due to their increased viscosity and relative absence of air bubbles. In addition, it is likely that cavitation will disrupt whole cells, causing cell death before DNA degradation.

16.3.3 Cells in Suspension

Again it appears that cavitation is required for observable cell damage. The effects observed are cell lysis, change in membrane permeabilities, e.g. loss of potassium ions from cells and damage to cell organelles, observed by electron microscopy and suggesting the possibility of cavitation nuclei within the cells. There appears to be little, if any, loss in reproductive ability. In general, cells which survive insonation can go on to reproduce normally.

There has obviously been considerable interest (as a result of the known effects of ionising radiation) in the genetic effects of ultrasound and experiments have been carried out to try and detect chromosome breakage, which in fact does not seem to occur even at very high intensities. Another effect which has been noted with chemical mutagens and investigated using ultrasound is sister chromatid exchange (SCE). Just before a cell divides the chromosomes double, giving rise to sister chromatids, and these can break and re-join but with a swap of identical chromatid segments between sisters. There is thus no change in genetic sequence and no mutagenic effect and in fact this process occurs naturally, but there is an increase in the frequency at which it occurs at low levels of chemicals which, at higher levels, are noticeably mutagenic. The effect can be detected under a microscope using staining techniques which allow the sister chromatids to be differentiated and exchanged chromatid segments identified (Figure 16.15).

As with many other potential effects, sister chromatid exchange following exposure to ultrasound has been reported but not independently verified.

16.3.4 Tissues

It is known from experiments on heating tissues that histological changes result from a sustained

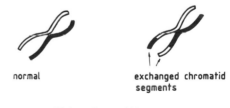

normal   exchanged chromatid segments

Sister Chromatids

Figure 16.15 Sister chromatid exchange.

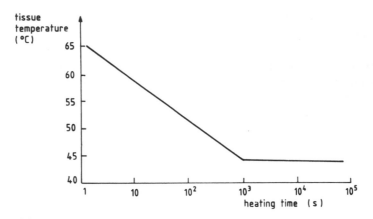

Figure 16.16 Duration of heating required to kill brain cells. Reproduced, with permission, from Lele, P.P. (1977) Thresholds and mechanisms of ultrasonic damage to organised animal tissues. In: W.G. Hazzard and M. Litz (eds) *Symposium on Biological Effects and Characterizations of Ultrasound Sources*, pp. 224–239. Hew Publication (FDA) 78–8048.

temperature of 44–45°C, or higher for short-duration heating (Figure 16.16), although the threshold temperature will depend to a certain degree on the tissue type.

As we have seen during insonation with ultrasound, the equilibrium temperature depends not only on the intensity but also on the duty cycle, the volume insonated and the blood supply to the tissue. Tissues with a poor blood supply (e.g. cornea) are expected to be especially susceptible. In fact, it is noted that in well-perfused tissue, the blood perfusion increases as the temperature rises during insonation, there being an approximately 2–3 times increase in muscle blood perfusion as the temperature is raised to 40–45°C.

Obviously, strongly attenuating tissues will have a greater rise in temperature and it is observed that bone, being a particularly strong attenuator, has a higher temperature rise than soft tissue under similar circumstances.

There is a reversible, followed by an irreversible (at higher intensities), blocking of nerve conduction when nerves are insonated with ultrasound and it is thought that this process has a thermal origin.

As we have seen previously, there is the potential for mode conversion followed by local soft tissue heating at a soft tissue–bone interface, and this heating of the periosteum is thought to be a cause of pain at high physiotherapy levels.

16.3.5 Streaming

It is thought that ultrasound-induced streaming of the blood is a cause of the endothelial damage observed in chick embryo and mouse uterine blood vessels since there is no damage at these levels to nearby tissues. It should be noted that endothelial damage occurs naturally and there are mechanisms for endothelial replacement. Permanent damage has not been demonstrated.

In some plant tissues, streaming and rotation of structures close to intercellular gas has been demonstrated at quite low levels of ultrasound, but no irreversible effects demonstrated below 3.5 W/cm². In some plants without natural gas spaces, 35 W/cm² are required to produce the same effect observed at 350 mW/cm² in space-containing tissues.

16.3.6 Cavitation

The evidence for cavitation occurring in whole tissues is that holes have been seen in excised mammalian tissue after insonation at a few watts per square centimetre at 1 MHz, but not at higher frequencies at the same power level.

An 8-MHz B-scan imager has been used to image small bubbles in guinea pig legs after insonation at 80 mW/cm², and above, at a frequency of 1.75 MHz. The bubbles disappeared when the ambient pressure was increased.

16.3.7 Standing Wave Effects

Stationary banding of red blood cells in chick embryo blood vessels within a standing wave field has been demonstrated (Figure 16.17). This could possibly lead to a reduction in cell flow and therefore oxygen deprivation if a standing wave field is set up between a transducer and a strong reflector (e.g. bone) for several minutes.

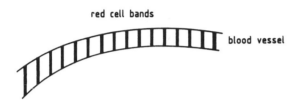

Figure 16.17 Red cell banding in a standing wave field.

16.3.8 Therapy Ultrasound

Therapy ultrasound levels are in the range 0.125–3.0 W/cm² SATA at low megahertz frequencies and the aim is to produce non-destructive beneficial biological effects. It is used as a method of deep heat delivery, the high absorption by large protein molecules meaning that collagenous tissues are preferentially heated. The effects are an increase in tendon extensibility, a decrease in joint stiffness, pain relief (poorly understood) and a decrease in muscle spasm thought to be the effect of temperature on nerve endings. As we have noted, there is also an increase in blood perfusion in muscle by a factor of approximately 2–3 following heating to 40–45°C, leading to an improvement of oxygen and nutrient supply and waste removal from tissues.

Possible non-thermal effects in physiotherapy are so-called micromassage due to the cyclical pressure variation which may help in loosening adhesions in soft tissue injuries, and acoustic streaming causing an alteration in biomolecule concentration gradients around membranes which may aid the diffusion processes involved in tissue injury repair.

16.3.9 Acceleration of Wound Healing

There are three main phases of wound healing:

(1) The inflammatory phase in which there is phagocytic activity by macrophages and leucocytes followed by digestion of material by lysosomal enzymes from macrophages.
(2) The proliferative phase in which there is a migration of cells to the wound region, plus rapid division and collagen synthesis by fibroblasts.
(3) Remodelling in which scar tissue is formed by the laying down of collagen fibres.

It is known that there is an acceleration of wound healing at ultrasound levels of 0.1–0.5 W/cm² and it is thought that the observed effect on lysosomal membranes in the inflammatory phase, an increase in protein synthesis by fibroblasts irradiated *in vitro*, and the observed increase in elasticity and strength of scar tissue in the remodelling phase are elements in this observed improvement.

There is an improvement in bone repair when ultrasound is used during the inflammatory and early proliferative stages, leading to direct ossification and little cartilage production, but not when insonation takes place in the late proliferative stage, in which unwanted cartilage production is actually stimulated. Since lower frequencies appear to be more effective than higher frequencies, a non-thermal effect is suggested.

16.3.10 Surgical Use

High-intensity (focussed) ultrasound is used for tissue destruction, for example in Meniere's disease.

16.3.11 Cancer Treatment

Tumour hyperthermia (heating to greater than 40°C) is a recognised method of tumour destruction and it is recognised that energy can be better localised with ultrasound than with the alternative of electromagnetic radiation. There is some evidence of a synergysm with X-rays and cytotoxic drugs but this evidence is equivocal.

16.3.12 Whole Body Effects

Investigation of whole body effects has concentrated on the fetus, firstly because it is known that a sustained increase in fetal temperature *in utero* of greater than 2.5°C can lead to increased abnormalities (it should be noted that increases of 0.4°C in the human uterus is quite normal) and also because it is easy to insonate the whole of a small mammal fetus. As expected, increased abnormalities at sustained therapeutic levels of ultrasound have been observed and the heating effect is probably involved.

16.3.13 Epidemiology

Epidemiological studies involve the examination of large samples of the population with both control and insonated groups to attempt to detect an effect of diagnostic ultrasound use. There are several problems involved in studies of this kind. Firstly, we are dealing with the comparatively low levels of intensity used in diagnostic imaging and the ultrasound beam is not stationary on any particular volume of tissue for very long, so any effect is likely to be very small. This means that extremely large numbers are required in the exposed and control groups. Groups of a few hundred are simply not able to demonstrate effects which may occur in a few cases every thousand patients. Secondly, it is important to have comparable exposed and control groups, since other factors such as socio-economic status may have an effect on fetal survival and birthweight, for example. Thirdly, since

ultrasound is so widely used now, it is in fact difficult to find unexposed control groups. The studies have concentrated on fetal abnormalities because of the understandable interest in this area, the known susceptibility of the first trimester fetus and the large number of obstetric scans carried out.

Investigators have looked for changes in the percentage of low-birthweight babies, the number of cases of childhood cancer, malformation and developmental problems. A number of studies have been carried out and no statistically significant differences between exposed and control groups have been found.

16.4 POWER AND INTENSITY MEASUREMENT

16.4.1 Significance of Intensity Measurements

Referring back to Section 2.3.2, we can see that the intensities most likely to be involved with thermal effects are those averaged over time. The highest time average intensity in the beam is given by I_{spta} and this will be of importance with stationary beams (e.g. Doppler examinations). I_{sata} is likely to be the intensity most related to thermal effects with scanned beams. On the other hand, non-linear effects and transient cavitation rely on high-pulse pressure and the quantities I_{sptp} and peak negative pressure are of interest here.

16.4.2 Power Measurement

Power output from a transducer can be measured using calorimetry, by radiation balance and, indirectly, by hydrophone.

16.4.2.1 Calorimetry

This is illustrated in Figure 16.18. Ultrasound from a transducer is completely absorbed within a material (usually a fluid such as castor oil or carbon tetrachloride). The initial rate of

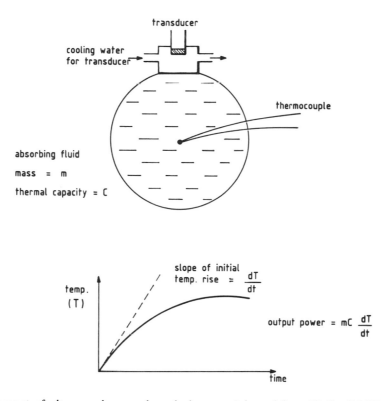

Figure 16.18 Measurement of ultrasound power by calorimetry. Adapted from Wells, P.N.T. *et al.* (1963) The dosimetry of small ultrasonic beams. *Ultrasonics*, **1**, 106–110. By permission of the publishers, Butterworth & Co. (Publishers) Ltd. ©.

temperature rise after switching on the ultrasound can be used to calculate the power output of the transducer. It is easier to measure the larger temperature rises obtained at higher power levels.

16.4.2.2 Radiation Force Measurement

In this method the force on a reflector or absorber due to the radiation from a transducer is measured and the relationship between force and power output used (see Section 16.2.2). Typical radiation balances are illustrated in Figure 16.19. It is important to avoid standing wave patterns being set up and their presence can be detected by moving the transducer along the beam axis and noting any change in reading. Streaming may also affect the radiation balance measurement and efforts have been made to reduce this effect

by the inclusion of a thin membrane between the transducer and the reflector or absorber. It is important to make sure that the transmission through this membrane is high and that no standing wave patterns are set up by virtue of its inclusion. Balances involving suspension wires passing out of the water into air are subject to varying surface tension forces on the wire and account has to be taken of this during measurement. This clearly does not affect balances contained completely within the water. Changes in water temperature can affect the buoyancy of the balance components so that it is important that the balance reaches an equilibrium temperature after each measurement and care is taken to avoid excessive heating due to absorption of the ultrasound and heat from the transducer itself.

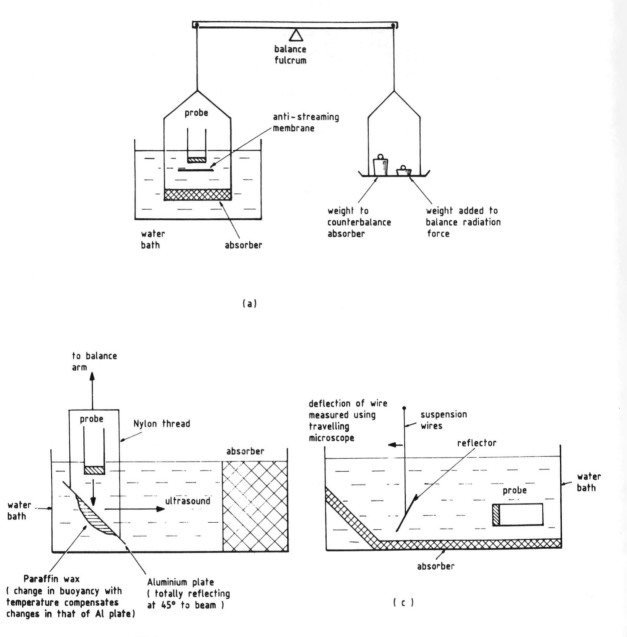

Figure 16.19 Radiation balances. Perpendicular absorber (a), angled reflector (b), horizontal deflection (c) and totally immersed balance (d). (a) adapted, with permission, from Williams, A.R. (1983) *Ultrasound: Biological Effects and Potential Hazards*, Academic Press. (b) reproduced, with permission, from Hill, C.R. (1970) Calibration of ultrasonic beams for biomedical applications. *Physics in Medicine and Biology*, **15**, 241–248. (c) adapted, with permission, from Woodcock, J.P. (1979) *Ultrasonics*, Adam Hilger, Ltd. (d) reproduced from Well, P.N.T. *et al.* (1963) The dosimetry of small ultrasonic beams. *Ultrasonics*, **1**, 106–110. By permission of the publishers, Butterworth & Co. (Publishers) Ltd. ©.

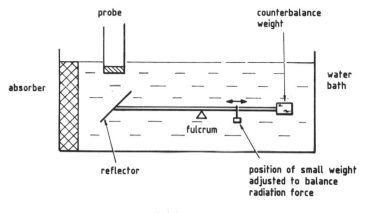

(d)

Figure 16.19 (*Continued*).

16.4.3 Hydrophones and Intensity Measurement

The previous two methods measure total power output, and in order to calculate intensities, we need a measurement of pulse and beam shape. A hydrophone is a small transducer which is used to measure local excess pressure strengths as illustrated in Figure 16.20. The output of the hydrophone is noted as it is moved throughout the beam, and by plotting the output voltage against position, the excess pressure variation in the beam can be plotted. Typical plots are shown in Figure 16.21.

Referring back to Sections 2.2.5 and 2.3.2 we see that intensities can be calculated from the pressure measurements. I_{sptp} is calculated from the peak of the pressure pulse (pulse amplitude) at the position of its highest value in the beam. The spacial peak intensity may be averaged over the pulse length to give I_{sppa} (spacial peak, pulse average) and this used to calculate the temporal average:

$$I_{spta} = \frac{\tau_p}{T_p} I_{sppa} \qquad (16.7)$$

where τ_p = the pulse length
and T_p = the pulse repetition period
(1/PRF)

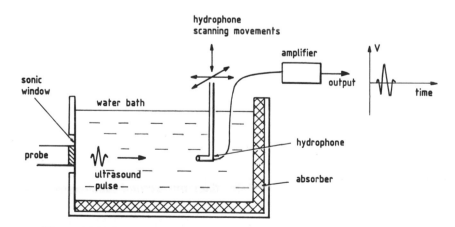

Figure 16.20 Measurement of an ultrasound field using a hydrophone.

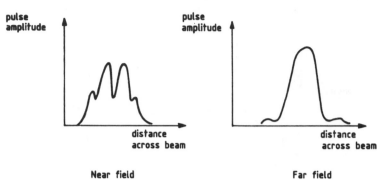

Figure 16.21 Cross-beam pulse pressure amplitude variation in the near and far field.

The total power (W) in the ultrasound beam can be found by adding the temporal average intensity contributions at all points over the beam cross-section. The spacial average intensity is then calculated from:

$$I_{\text{sata}} = W/A \qquad (16.8)$$

where A is the beam cross-sectional area calculated from the beam diameter measured from the pressure amplitude plots.

This calculation of total power also enables the hydrophone to be calibrated against radiation balance measurements.

The structure of a small PZT hydrophone is shown in Figure 16.22. The structure of a membrane hydrophone is shown in Figure 16.23. Hydrophones with very small sensitive areas and therefore capable of high resolution can be constructed using this technique. A multi-channel membrane hydrophone is shown in Figure 16.24. This consists of a number of independent hydrophones formed on a single membrane and which, placed across an ultrasound beam, can indicate the pressure variation without resort to scanning.

16.5 SAFETY

16.5.1 Recommended Levels

In 1982 the American Institute of Ultrasound in Medicine (AIUM) issued the following pronouncement in safety:

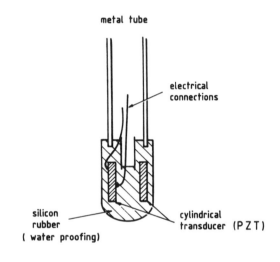

Figure 16.22 PZT hydrophone construction. Reproduced, with permission, from Hill, C.R. (1970) Calibration of ultrasonic beams for biomedical applications. *Physics in Medicine and Biology*, **15(2)**, 241–248.

In the low MHz frequency range, there have been no independently confirmed significant biological effects in mammalian tissues exposed to intensities (SPTA as measured in a free-field of water) below 100 milliwatts per square centimeter. Furthermore, for ultrasonic exposure times less than 500 seconds and greater than one second, such effects have not been demonstrated even at higher intensities, when the product of intensity and exposure time is less than 50 Joules per cm².

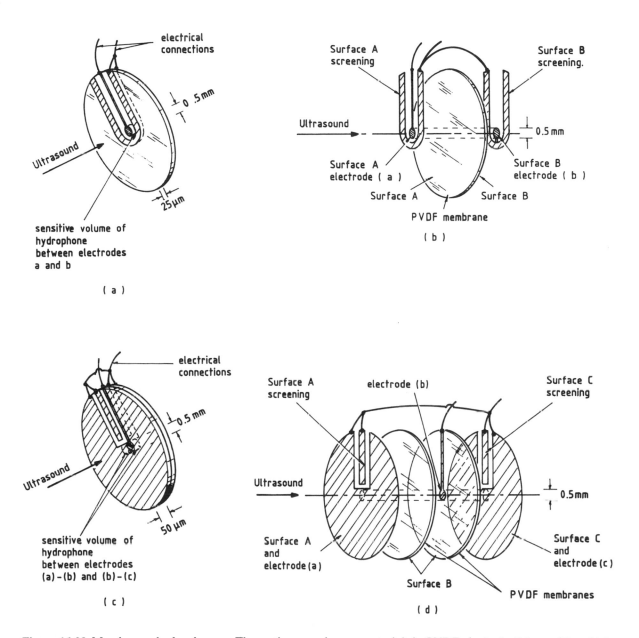

Figure 16.23 Membrane hydrophones. The active membrane material is PVDF (polyvinylidene difluoride). Coplanar (single membrane) hydrophone construction (a). Exploded view (b). The transducer or active volume of the hydrophone is a short cylinder between electrodes (a) and (b). Bilaminar (double membrane) hydrophone construction (c). Exploded view (d). Electrical screening from outside interference is improved by the use of large 'ground' electrodes on the outer surfaces (A and C). The sensitive volume of the hydrophone consists of two short cylindrical transducers between electrodes (b) and (a) and between electrodes (b) and (c). It is effectively two transducers connected in series, the polarity of the two being in opposite directions such that their electrical outputs add when they are connected as shown. Reproduced by permission of Dr. R. Preston. Crown copyright.

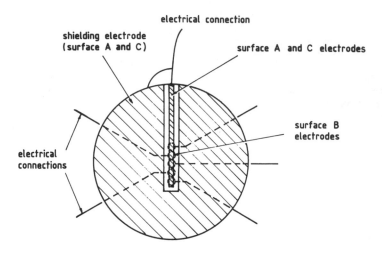

Each hydrophone is formed between a surface B electrode and the common electrodes on surface A and C.

Figure 16.24 Multi-channel, bilaminar membrane hydrophone construction. Reproduced by permission of Dr. R. Preston. Crown copyright.

From this statement we can infer limits of

$$I_{spta} < 100 \text{ mW/cm}^2$$

$$I_{spta} \times \text{Time} < 50 \text{ J cm}^2$$

$$\text{For } 1 \text{ s} > \text{Time} > 500 \text{ s}$$

In 1987 the AIUM issued a similar statement for unfocussed ultrasound but also stated that the effects had not been demonstrated for focussed ultrasound where I_{spta} was less than 1 W/cm².

It has been realised that the intensity of the ultrasound measured in water is an overestimate of the intensity at the same depth in tissue, as a result of the higher attenuation of tissue. In addition, it is thought that the differing sensitivity of tissues to ultrasound should be taken into account when recommending maximum levels. The Federal Drug Administration (FDA) recommended maximum values for I_{spta} *in situ* and in water for different types of examination and these are shown in Table 16.1.

The most recent recommendation of the British Medical Ultrasound Society Working Party on the 'Prudent use of Diagnostic Ultrasound' is that the earlier 1982 AIUM recommended limits should be adhered to.

Table 16.1 Food and Drug Administration (USA) recommended maximum intensities.

Use	I_{spta} in situ (mW/cm²)	I_{spta} in water (mW/cm²)
Cardiac	430	730
Peripheral vessel	720	1500
Opthalmic	17	68
Fetal imaging and other*	94	180

*Abdominal, intraoperative, paediatric, small organ (breast, thyroid, testes), cephalic.

16.5.2 Output Levels

The problem of recommended maximum levels is complicated by the fact that recent surveys of the output of commercial ultrasound instruments have shown a wide range of output powers (Table 16.2). The maximum power from some instruments is well above the limit and the pulsed Doppler beams from some duplex scanners can have extremely high output powers.

The AIUM 1982 recommended levels in a graphical form, together with a rough indication

Table 16.2 Output levels from surveys of commercial diagnostic instruments.

	Min.	Max.
Imagers (arrays and mechanical sector scanners)		
I_{spta} (mW/cm^2)	0.02	440
I_{sppa} (mW/cm^2)	110	720 000
Peak negative pressure (MPa)	0.04	0.65
Pulsed Doppler		
I_{spta} (mW/cm^2)	40	4000
I_{sppa} (mW/cm^2)	280	150 000
Peak negative pressure (Pa)	0.1	1.55

Reproduced with permission from Blackwell, R. (1988) *Safety of diagnostic ultrasound.* In: R. A. Lerski (ed.) *Practical Ultrasound*, p. 235, IRL Press.

of the diagnostic ultrasound zone and its extension due to the new higher power instruments, are shown in Figure 16.25.

It should be noted that there is now a considerable overlap between the intensity levels used for therapy and those used for imaging. Since the aim of therapeutic ultrasound is to produce a biological effect and effects have been demonstrated in the 'therapeutic range', it is clear that some effect may be expected from the now high diagnostic levels. It should be particularly noted that the use of pulsed Doppler requires the ultrasound beam to be maintained in a single position for a much longer time than is normally used for imaging, so giving an increased exposure to the tissues within the beam.

16.5.3 Benefit/Risk Judgement

The decision on whether to use ultrasound and the levels to be used reduces to a benefit/risk judgement. That is to say, the benefit likely to accrue to a patient by carrying out an examination needs to be balanced against the risk of that particular examination.

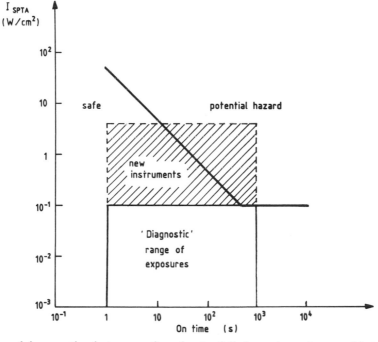

Figure 16.25 The line of demarcation between safe and potentially hazardous ultrasound intensities and durations inferred from the AIUM 1982 statement.

16.5.4 Safety Rules*

Some broad rules can be formulated to protect against unnecessary exposure to ultrasound. These are as follows:

(1) Do not scan unless there is a clear clinical objective.
(2) Have regular instrument checks.
(3) Discover if the ultrasound output is disabled when frame freeze is used. It not, remove the probe when making measurements from the screen.
(4) Use the output attenuator to reduce the transmitted power to the minimum level consistent with the required image quality.
(5) If the output of the instrument exceeds 100 mW/cm², calculate the time you can dwell on one point before the 50 J/cm² limit is exceeded.
(6) Take special care when scanning sensitive organs (e.g. early pregnancy, eye, gonads) and when microbubbles are introduced into the beam (e.g. oocyte recovery) since these may reduce the cavitation threshold.
(7) Keep up to date on scanning techniques so that patients get maximum value for minimum exposure.
(8) Do not allow trainee radiographers too much time on any one patient.
(9) Keep up to date on recommended levels of exposure and hazard.

*Reproduced, with permission, from Blackwell, R. (1988) Safety of diagnostic ultrasound. In: R. A. Lerski (ed.) *Practical Ultrasound*, p. 238, IRL Press.

APPENDIX A

Maths Notes

A.1 EXPONENTS

A.1.1 Definition

If n is the exponent of a then:

$$a^n = a \times a \times a \ldots n \text{ times}$$

A.1.2 Multiplication

$$a^n \times a^m = a^{n+m}$$

e.g. $2^3 \times 2^2 = 2^5 = 32$

A.1.3 Division

$$a^n/a^m = a^{n-m}$$

e.g. $2^3/2^2 = 2^1 = 2$

A.1.4 Reciprocal

$$a^{-m} = 1/a^m$$

e.g. $2^{-2} = 1/2^2 = 0.25$

A.1.5 Zero Exponent

$$a^0 = 1$$

since $1 = a^n/a^n = a^{n-n} = a^0$

A.1.6 Powers of 10

Millionth	$\dfrac{1}{1\,000\,000}$	0.000001	10^{-6}
	$\dfrac{1}{100\,000}$	0.00001	10^{-5}
	$\dfrac{1}{10\,000}$	0.0001	10^{-4}
Thousandth	$\dfrac{1}{1000}$	0.001	10^{-3}
Hundredth	$\dfrac{1}{100}$	0.01	10^{-2}
Tenth	$\dfrac{1}{10}$	0.1	10^{-1}
	1	1	10^{0}
Ten	10		10^{1}
Hundred	100		10^{2}
Thousand	1000		10^{3}
Ten thousand	10\,000		10^{4}
Hundred thousand	100\,000		10^{5}
Million	1\,000\,000		10^{6}

A.2 TRIGONOMETRIC (TRIG) FUNCTIONS

$\cos \theta = A/H$

$\sin \theta = O/H$

$\tan \theta = O/A$

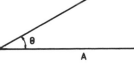

221

A.3 LOGARITHMS (LOGS)

A.3.1 Definition (of log of x)

$$x = 10^{(\log (x))}$$

Note that this is the definition of the most common (base 10 or Naperian) logarithm. Logarithms may be defined for other bases and to avoid confusion the base is sometimes noted as a subscript. Thus the logarithm defined above may be written $\log_{10}(x)$.

A.3.2 Properties

The log of the product of two numbers is the sum of their logs:

$$\log (xy) = \log (x) + \log (y)$$

since $xy = 10^{\log (x)} \times 10^{\log (y)}$
$= 10^{(\log (x) - \log (y))}$

The log of the quotient of two numbers is the difference of their logs:

$$\log (x/y) = \log (x) - \log (y)$$

since $x/y = 10^{\log (x)}/10^{\log (y)} = 10^{(\log (x) - \log (y))}$

APPENDIX B

DeciBel (dB) Scale

B.1 INTRODUCTION

The deciBel scale is a way of expressing the ratios of intensities or powers. Its advantages lie in its being a logarithmic scale. Firstly, it compresses the wide range of intensities and powers found in practice into a relatively small (and more manageable) range of numbers. Secondly, products of ratios encountered when dealing with attenuation in different layers of tissue and successive stages in a signal progression through an instrument may be evaluated by adding the deciBel representations of these ratios.

B.2 DEFINITION

Intensity ratio (dB) $= 10 \log_{10} (I/I_0)$ dB

Signal (power) ratio (dB) $= 10 \log_{10} (P/P_0)$ dB

Since the power in an electrical circuit is proportional to voltage squared, the above may be written (where voltages V and V_0 correspond to powers P and P_0):

Signal ratio (dB) $= 10 \log_{10} (V/V_0)^2$ dB

$= 20 \log_{10} (V/V_0)$ dB

which follows from the properties of logarithms.

B.3 EXAMPLES

B.3.1 dB Level

If I_0 or P_0 are fixed reference levels then intensity or power levels can be quoted in dB. If we set a reference level of 1 mW/cm^2 then an intensity of 100 mW/cm^2 is $10 \log_{10} (100) = 20$ dB.

B.3.2 Attenuation

Since attenuation reduces intensity, leading to $I/I_0 < 1$ and a negative logarithm, it is usual to express attenuation as:

Atten $= -10 \log_{10} (I/I_0)$ dB

If passage through a layer of tissue reduces the intensity of ultrasound from 100 mW/cm^2 to 10 mW/cm^2 then the attenuation is:

Atten$_1 = -10 \log_{10} (10/100)$ dB

$= 10$ dB

If passage through a further layer reduces the intensity from 10 mW/cm^2 to 2 mW/cm^2 then the attenuation in this further layer is:

Atten$_2 = -10 \log_{10} (2/10)$ dB

$= 7$ dB

The overall attenuation is:

$$\text{Atten}_3 = \text{Atten}_1 + \text{Atten}_2$$
$$= 17 \text{ dB}$$

B.3.3 Gain

If the voltage input to an amplifier is V_{in} and the output V_{out} then its gain is:

$$\text{Gain} = 20 \log_{10} (V_{out}/V_{in}) \text{ dB}$$

A preamplifier which boosts a signal from 10 μV to 300 μV has a gain of:

$$G_1 = 20 \log_{10} (300/10) \text{ dB}$$
$$= 29.5 \text{ dB}$$

The amplifier following this has a voltage gain of 200. Its gain on the dB scale is:

$$G_2 = 20 \log_{10} (200) \text{ dB}$$
$$= 46 \text{ dB}$$

The overall gain is:

$$G = G_2 + G_2 = 75.5 \text{ dB}$$

B.4 TABLE OF VALUES

I/I_0	dB
10^{10}	100
10^6	60
10^2	20
10	10
2	3
1	0
0.5	−3
10^{-1}	−10
10^{-2}	−20
10^{-6}	−60
10^{-10}	−100

B.5 ATTENUATION COEFFICIENT

The ratio of the intensity, at depth x in material with attenuation coefficient α, to the incident intensity I_0 is:

$$I/I_0 = e^{-\alpha x}$$

On the dB scale:

$$10 \log_{10} (I/I_0) = 10 \log_{10} (e^{-\alpha x}) \text{ dB}$$
$$= -10\alpha \log_{10} (e)x \text{ dB}$$
$$= -4.3\alpha x \text{ dB}$$

This may be written:

$$10 \log_{10} (I/I_0) = -\mu x$$

where $\mu = -10 \log_{10} (I/I_0)/x$

= the dB attenuation coefficient in dB/n

and $\mu = 4.3\alpha$

If the attenuation coefficient is quoted in dB m^{-1} MHz^{-1} then this figure must be multiplied by the frequency (in MHz) to obtain μ (in dB/m) and this multiplied by 4.3 to obtain α.

Measurement Statistics

C.1 INTRODUCTION

Whenever we make a number of measurements of a physical quantity, we find that we do not get exactly the same answer each time. The differences are due to operator error, small random changes due to noise in the measurement system and changes between samples of the quantity we are trying to measure.

C.2 RESULTS HISTOGRAM

If we take a number of measurements of a quantity x, say, we can examine the spread of results by plotting them in a histogram form as shown in Figure C.1a. The height of each histogram bar represents the number of readings within a small range around the value of x at the mid-point of the bar. For example, the histogram shows that there were 25 readings lying between $x = 5.5$ and $x = 6.5$ and two between $x = 1.5$ and $x = 2.5$. The total number of readings (100) is the sum of the readings from each histogram bar range.

C.3 PROBABILITY HISTOGRAM

We may display these results in terms of probability (Figure C.1b). Since 25 out of 100 readings are between $x = 5.5$ and $x = 6.5$, the probability of finding a reading within this range is 25/100 or 0.25.

Note that when we add up all the probabilities, we get a value of one. That is to say, the probability of finding a result within the total range of results is one, or certainty. Note also that the probability represented by each histogram bar is proportional to the area of the bar and the probability of finding a reading between limits encompassing a number of histogram bars is the total area of those bars.

C.4 PROBABILITY DENSITY FUNCTION

If we increase the number of readings taken, we can decrease the width of the probability histogram bars and increase the number of points within each bar. Eventually, the histogram bars become sufficiently close that the outline is indistinguishable from a smooth curve, as shown in Figure C.1c. The probability of finding a reading within a small range Δx about x_1 is the hatched area and is equal to:

$$P_{\Delta x}(x_1) = P(x_1)\Delta x \qquad (C.1)$$

The function $P(x)$ is called a probability density function (PDF) and the most common shape of the graph of such a function describing measurement errors is the bell-shape shown. This is called a normal or Gaussian PDF.

C.5 MEAN AND STANDARD DEVIATION

If we take N readings $(x_1, x_2, x_3 \ldots$ etc.) of a quantity x, then the mean value of x is:

$$\bar{x} = (x_1 + x_2 + x_3 \ldots)/N \qquad (C.2)$$

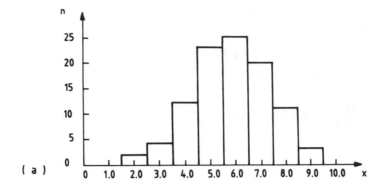

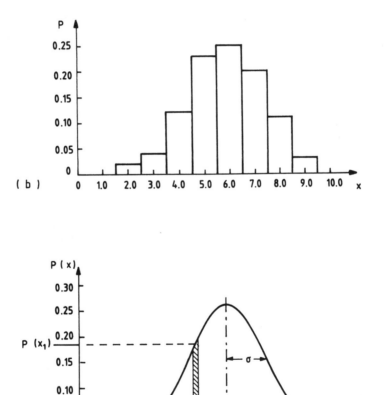

Figure C.1 Measurement results histogram (a), corresponding probability histogram (b) and Gaussian probability density function (c).

If all the errors are equally likely to be negative as positive, then $\bar{x}$ is an estimate of the value we are trying to measure and will get closer to this value as N increases. If the errors are more likely to be either positive or negative, then $\bar{x}$ will not get closer to the true value and the difference for large N is called the bias in the result.

The spread in the result is determined by first calculating the square of the deviations of each result from the mean value, calculating the mean value of these squared deviations and taking the square root to obtain a root-mean-square deviation (also called the standard deviation of the readings):

$$\text{Std dev.} = \sigma = \sqrt{\frac{x_1 - \bar{x})^2 + (x_2 - \bar{x})^2 + \ldots}{N}}$$

(C.3)

Since the calculated value of $\bar{x}$ for small N is likely to be significantly different from the limiting value for large N, the squared deviations in the above are overestimated and it is found that a more accurate estimate of the standard deviation is obtained by replacing N by $N - 1$ in equation C.2. The difference is, of course, negligible for large N.

The values of $\bar{x}$ and σ are indicated in Figure C.1c.

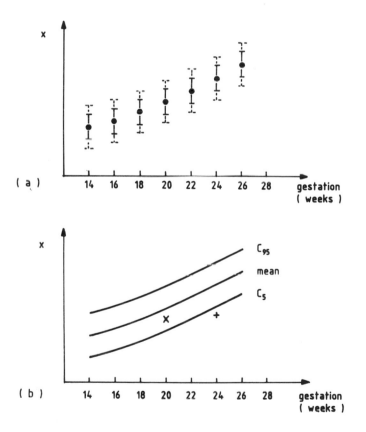

Figure C.2 The mean (point), plus and minus 1 standard deviation (solid bars) and 5 and 95 centile limits (dashed lines) of a typical fetal measurement at a range of gestational ages (a) and mean and normal range of the measurement taken from the above (b).

C.6 CENTILES

Another method of showing the spread of results is the position of the centiles. A centile is a value of x which indicates the upper limit enclosing a given percentage of the results. For example, the fifth centile C_5 is such that 5% of the results lie below it. This means that the cross-hatched area in Figure C.1c is 5% of the total area under the curve. The 95th centile C_{95} (also shown) is such that 95% of the results lie below it. We can see that 90% of the results lie between C_5 and C_{95} and that the probability of results lying outside these limits is small.

C.7 FETAL MEASUREMENTS

Measurements are made on the fetus in order to assess growth patterns and to detect growth retardation. Measurements include bi-parietal diameter, crown–rump length and abdominal circumference. If readings of a particular quantity are taken on a large number of fetuses at different gestational ages, then the results may be presented as shown in Figure C.2a. At each age the mean, plus and minus the standard deviation, and the 5th and 95th centiles, are shown. If the mean and the centiles are plotted using continuous lines (as shown in Figure C.2b) then we have a convenient method of checking fetal growth. Readings lying between the 5th and 95th centiles may be assumed within the normal range, whereas readings lying below the 5th centile have a high probability of indicating growth retardation. Sequential measurements allow assessment of the growth pattern.

Cathode Ray Tube (CRT) Display

D.1 THE CATHODE RAY TUBE

The diagram of the CRT is shown in Figure D.1a. An evacuated glass envelope contains a number of metal electrodes and a screen covered on the inside with a phosphor which emits light when bombarded with electrons. Electrons are emitted from an electrically heated cathode (C), attracted and accelerated towards the screen by a high positive potential with respect to the cathode on the cylindrical anodes A_1 and A_2. The two anodes form an electrostatic lens and by adjusting the potential between them the electron beam can be made to converge (focus) to a spot on the screen. Where the electrons hit the phosphor, light is emitted.

The spot is deflected to different parts of the screen by varying the potential difference across the deflection plates X_1X_2 and Y_1Y_2, shown from the screen end of the tube in Figure D.1b. A positive potential on vertical deflection plate Y_2 with respect to Y_1 attracts the electron beam, and therefore the light spot, upwards. Reversing the polarity will move the spot downwards. Similarly the spot can be moved horizontally, using the horizontal deflection electrodes X_1 and X_2.

An alternative (magnetic) method of beam deflection is shown in Figure D.1c. The electron beam is deflected by the magnetic field formed in the gap between opposing coils by passing a (deflection) current through the coils. The strength of the magnetic field and therefore the spot deflection depends on the current strength.

The force on the beam is perpendicular to the magnetic field and therefore the X and Y deflection coils are in the positions shown. This form of deflection is usually used in video monitors.

D.2 THE OSCILLOSCOPE

The oscilloscope uses a CRT to display time varying signals, for example the A-scan. The vertical and horizontal deflection electrodes of the CRT are connected as shown in Figure D.2a. The time varying signals to be displayed are amplified and applied to the vertical deflection plates, whereas a time base is connected to the horizontal deflection plates. The time base generates a series of voltage ramps as shown in Figure D.2b which move the spot at a constant speed across the screen. Thus, the horizontal position of the spot from its starting point is proportional to the elapsed time. The horizontal axis can be thought of as a time axis—hence the term 'time base'. The display (Figure D.2d) matches the time variation of the signal to be displayed (Figure D.2c).

D.3 THE VIDEO MONITOR

The spot on the screen of a video monitor is moved in a zig-zag or raster fashion as shown in Figure D.3. The spot is moved rapidly across the screen, using a fast (line) time base and more

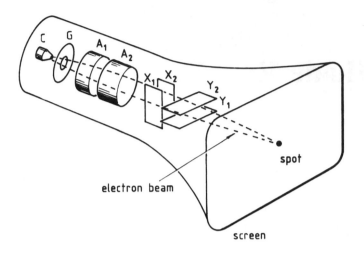

(a)

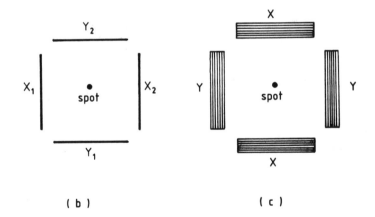

(b)   (c)

Figure D.1 The cathode ray tube (CRT) construction (a), and views of deflection plates (b) or deflection coils (c) from the screen looking towards the cathode.

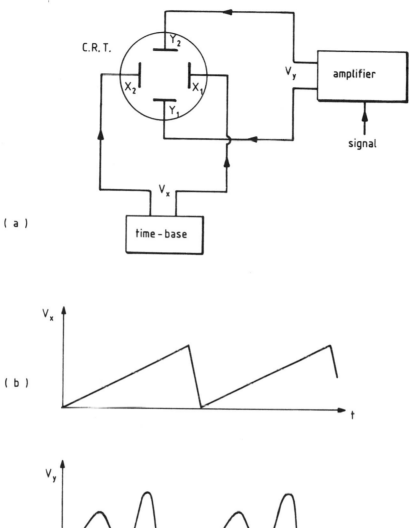

(a)

(b)

(c)

(d)

Figure D.2 The oscilloscope. Block diagram (a), time base waveform (b), input signal (c) and display (d).

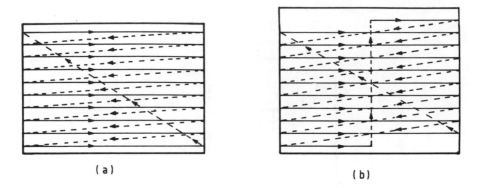

(a)   (b)

Figure D.3 The video raster scan. Simple (a) and interlaced (b).

slowly down the screen using a slower (frame) time base. In the simple raster scan (as shown in Figure D.3a) each of the horizontal lines is displayed in sequence. In the interlaced raster scan (as shown in Figure D.3b) the odd-numbered lines are displayed (counting from the top) followed by the even-numbered lines. Although more complex, the interlaced raster scan is more often used because the perception of flicker in the display is reduced since each line is followed by a line at half the total frame repetition period. The standard video raster pattern for the UK consists of 625 lines repeating at 25 frames per second, whereas in the USA the standard is 525 lines repeating at 30 frames per second.

The video signal supplied to video monitors contains synchronisation pulses to control the timing of the time bases and an intensity modulation signal to vary the brightness of the spot according to the position on the screen.

Filters

Filters are used to select signals within a certain frequency range from within a wider range of signal frequencies. The three types most commonly used in diagnostic ultrasound instruments are shown in Figure E.1.

The low-pass filter allows the passage of low-frequency signals and prevents the passage of high-frequency signals. The high-pass filter removes low frequencies and allows the passage of high frequencies whereas the band-pass filter allows the passage of the signal frequencies within a certain range.

As shown, the low-pass and high-pass filters are specified as having a certain cut-off frequency (f_{co}) whereas the band-pass filter is specified by a centre frequency (f_c) and bandwidth (BW).

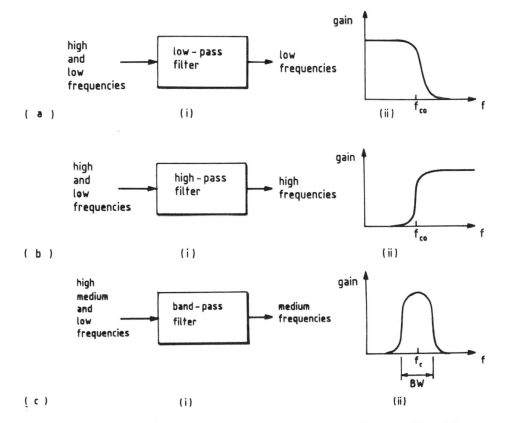

Figure E.1 Types of filter used in diagnostic ultrasound instruments. Filter type (i) and frequency response (ii). Low-pass filter (a), high-pass filter (b) and band-pass filter (c).

The Initial Rate of Temperature Rise in Insonated Tissue

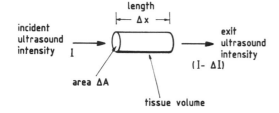

Figure F.1 Tissue volume geometry, and incident and exit ultrasound intensities for tissue heating calculation.

Consider the insonation of the small volume of tissue shown in Figure F.1.

By definition the attenuation coefficient is:

$$\alpha = \frac{1}{I}\frac{\Delta I}{\Delta x} \quad \text{nepers/m} \qquad \text{(F.1)}$$

for small Δx (strictly for $\dfrac{\Delta I}{I} \ll 1$)

where

$$\alpha = \underset{\text{(absorption)}}{\alpha_a} + \underset{\text{(scatter)}}{\alpha_s}$$

For most tissues $\alpha_s \ll \alpha_a$ and we can take $\alpha \simeq \alpha_a$.

The intensity loss in distance Δx is (from equation F.1):

$$\Delta I = I\alpha\Delta x \quad \text{W/m}^2$$

The power loss is therefore (power = intensity × area):

$$\Delta W = I\alpha\Delta x\Delta A$$
$$= I\alpha\Delta V \quad \text{W} \qquad \text{(F.2)}$$

where $\Delta V = \Delta x\Delta A$ = the volume of tissue.

But the power loss is the rate of loss of energy (by definition):

$$\Delta W = \frac{\Delta Q}{\Delta t} \quad \text{W (J/s)} \qquad \text{(F.3)}$$

where ΔQ is the loss of energy in time Δt.

Therefore (from equations F.2 and F.3) we have:

$$\frac{\Delta Q}{\Delta t} = I\alpha\Delta V \quad \text{J/s} \qquad \text{(F.4)}$$

Now if the tissue has a heat capacity C (heat energy in joules required to raise the temperature of 1 kg of tissue by 1°C) then our volume of tissue of mass $\rho\Delta V$ takes ΔQ J of energy to raise its temperature by ΔT°C where:

$$\Delta Q = \rho\Delta VC\Delta T \quad \text{J} \qquad \text{(F.5)}$$

Substituting for ΔQ from equation F.5 into equation F.4, and rearranging, gives the rate at which the tissue volume rises in temperature:

$$\frac{\Delta T}{\Delta t} = \frac{I\alpha}{\rho C} \quad \text{°C/s} \qquad \text{(F.6)}$$

For example, if: and $I = 10^4 \text{ W/m}^2 \ (1 \text{ W/cm}^2)$

$\alpha = 60 \text{ m}^{-1}$ (e.g. liver at 3 MHz)

$\rho = 10^3 \text{ kg/m}^3$ then $\dfrac{\Delta T}{\Delta t} = 0.14°\text{C/s}$

$C = 4.2 \times 10^3 \text{ J kg}^{-1} \, °\text{C}^{-1}$ or 8.6°C/min

Definitions of Some Fundamental Quantities

Acoustic Power
Rate of emission of energy from a source, or rate of transfer of energy across a surface.

Attenuation Coefficient
Rate of fractional decrease of intensity with distance.

Characteristic Acoustic Impedance
Ratio of excess pressure to particle velocity in a medium.

Energy
Capacity to do work.

Excess Pressure
Change in pressure in a medium resulting from the passage of an ultrasonic wave.

Frequency
Number of complete cycles of a wave motion, observed at a fixed point, per unit time.

Particle Velocity
Velocity of a particle of a medium due to the passage of a wave or pulse.

Period
Duration of a complete cycle of a wave observed at a fixed point.

Speed of Propagation
Distance travelled by a wave motion per unit time.

Tissue Compressibility
Ratio of fractional change in a volume of tissue to the excess pressure causing the change.

Tissue Density
Mass per unit volume of tissue.

Tissue Elastic Modulus
Ratio of the excess pressure to the fractional change in volume caused by the excess pressure.

Ultrasound Intensity
Power transferred through unit area perpendicular to the wave.

Wave Amplitude
Difference between maximum and resting values of oscillating quantity (e.g. pressure, particle displacement).

Wavelength
Distance between similar points on consecutive cycles of a wave observed at a fixed time.

Units

Scaling Prefix

Quantity	Units
Acoustic impedance	kg m^{-2}s^{-1}, rayls
Angle	degrees
Area	m^2
Attenuation coefficient α	m^{-1}
Attenuation coefficient μ	dB m^{-1}
Compliance	kg^{-1} m s^2
Density	kg m^{-3}
Elastic modulus	kg m^{-1} s^{-2}
Energy	joules (J)
Force	newtons (N)
Frequency	s^{-1}, hertz (Hz)
Intensity	W m^{-2}
Length	metre (m)
Mass	kilogram (kg)
Period	s
Power	J s^{-1}, watts (W)
Pressure	N m^{-2}, pascal (Pa)
Speed	m s^{-1}
Temperature	degrees Centigrade (°C)
Thermal capacity	J kg^{-1} °C^{-1}
Time	second (s)
Volume	m^3
Volume	litre (l) (1 l = 10^{-3} m^3)
Volume flow rate	l s^{-1}
Wavelength	m

Prefix	Name	Scaling
μ	micro-	millionth
m	milli-	thousandth
c	centi-	hundredth
k	kilo-	thousand
M	mega-	million

e.g. 5 MHz = 5 000 000 Hz
    4 mm = 0.004 m

APPENDIX I

Calculation Examples

I.1 FREQUENCY (f), WAVELENGTH (λ), SPEED (c)

Equation:

$$\lambda f = c \qquad (I.1)$$

Question 1:

Given $c = 1540$ m/s and $f = 1$ MHz what is λ?

Answer:

$$\lambda = c/f \qquad (I.2)$$
$$= 1540/10^6 \text{ m}$$
$$= 1.54 \times 10^{-3} \text{ m}$$
$$= 1.54 \text{ mm}$$

Question 2:

Given $c = 1540$ m/s and $\lambda = 0.3$ mm, what is f?

Answer:

$$\lambda = 0.3 \text{ mm}$$
$$= 0.3 \times 10^{-3} \text{ m}$$
$$f = c/\lambda \qquad (I.3)$$
$$= 1540/(0.3 \times 10^{-3}) \text{ Hz}$$
$$= 5.13 \times 10^6 \text{ Hz}$$
$$= 5.13 \text{ MHz}$$

I.2 REFLECTOR DEPTH (L), PULSE RETURN TIME (τ), SPEED (c)

Equation:

$$L = \frac{c\tau}{2} \qquad (I.4)$$

Question:

Given $c = 1540$ m/s and $L = 10$ cm what is τ?

Answer:

$$L = 10 \text{ cm}$$
$$= 0.1 \text{ m}$$
$$\tau = \frac{2L}{c} \qquad (I.5)$$
$$= \frac{0.2}{1540} \text{ s}$$
$$= 1.30 \times 10^{-4} \text{ s}$$
$$= 130 \text{ } \mu\text{s}$$

I.3 PULSE REPETITION FREQUENCY (PRF), MAXIMUM DEPTH (L_{max}), SPEED (c)

Equation:

$$PRF = \frac{c}{2L_{max}} \qquad (I.6)$$

Question:

Given $c = 1540$ m/s and $L_{max} = 20$ cm what is PRF?

Answer:

$$L_{max} = 20 \text{ cm}$$

$$= 0.2 \text{ m}$$

$$\text{PRF} = \frac{c}{2L_{max}}$$

$$\text{PRF} = \frac{1540}{0.4} \text{ Hz}$$

$$= 3850 \text{ Hz}$$

$$= 3.85 \text{ kHz}$$

I.4 FRAME RATE (f_r), PULSE REPETITION FREQUENCY (PRF), NUMBER OF SCAN LINES (N_s)

Equation:

$$f_r = \text{PRF}/N_s \qquad (I.7)$$

Question:

Given PRF = 7 kHz and $f_r = 20$ Hz what is N_s?

Answer:

$$N_s = \text{PRF}/f_r$$

$$= \frac{7000}{20}$$

$$= 350$$

I.5 FRAME RATE (f_r), MAXIMUM DEPTH (L_{max}), SPEED (c), BEAM SEPARATION, SCAN SIZE

Equation:

Eliminating PRF from I.6 and I.7 gives:

$$f_r = \frac{c}{2N_s L_{max}} \qquad (I.8)$$

Question:

Given a sector scanner with $L_{max} = 10$ cm, $f_r \simeq 30$ Hz, $c = 1540$ m/s and a beam separation of $0.25°$ what is the sector size?

Answer:

$$L_{max} = 10 \text{ cm}$$

$$= 0.1 \text{ m}$$

From equation I.8:

$$N_s = \frac{c}{2f_r L_{max}} \qquad (I.9)$$

$$= \frac{1540}{2 \times 30 \times 0.1}$$

$$= 256.7$$

To the nearest integer

$$N_s = 257$$

The number of intervals between the beams is 256.

Thus the sector size $= 256 \times 0.25°$

$$= 64°$$

I.6 ACOUSTIC IMPEDANCE (Z), INTENSITY REFLECTION COEFFICIENT (R)

Equation:

$$R = \left[\frac{Z_2 - Z_1}{Z_1 + Z_2} \right]^2 \qquad (I.10)$$

where Z_2 and Z_1 are the acoustic impedances either side of the reflecting interface.

Question:

Given $Z_1 = 1.38 \times 10^6$ rayl (fat) and $Z_2 = 1.70 \times 10^6$ rayl (muscle) what is R for a muscle–fat interface?

Answer:

$$R = \left[\frac{Z_2 - Z_1}{Z_1 + Z_2}\right]^2$$

$$= \left[\frac{1.70 - 1.38}{1.70 + 1.38}\right]^2$$

$$= 0.0108$$

$$\doteq 1.08\%$$

I.7 LENGTH OF NEAR ZONE (Z_m), TRANSDUCER DIAMETER (D), FREQUENCY (f), SPEED OF ULTRASOUND (c)

Equation:

$$Z_m = a^2/\lambda \qquad (I.11)$$

where a = transducer radius.
  Substituting $D = 2a$ gives

$$Z_m = \frac{D^2}{4\lambda} \qquad (I.12)$$

Eliminating λ from equations I.12 and I.1 gives

$$Z_m = \frac{D^2 f}{4c} \qquad (I.13)$$

Question:
Given D = 1.5 cm, f = 3.5 Mz and c = 1540 m/s what is Z_m?
Answer:

$$D = 1.5 \text{ cm}$$

$$= 0.015 \text{ m}$$

$$Z_m = \frac{0.015^2 \times 3.5 \times 10^6}{4 \times 1540} \text{ m}$$

$$= 0.128 \text{ m}$$

$$= 12.8 \text{ cm}$$

I.8 DEVIATION OF THE TRANSMITTED BEAM AT AN INTERFACE, ANGLE OF INCIDENCE (θ_i), SPEED OF ULTRASOUND (c)

Equation:

$$\frac{\sin \theta_t}{\sin \theta_i} = \frac{c_2}{c_1} \qquad (I.14)$$

where the quantities are defined in Figure 3.2.
Question:
Given c_2 = 1580 m/s (muscle), c_1 = 1450 m/s (fat) and θ_i = 30° what is the beam deviation ($\theta_t - \theta_i$) at a fat–muscle interface?
Answer:

$$\sin \theta_t = \frac{c_2}{c_1} \sin \theta_i$$

$$= \frac{1580}{1450} \sin 30°$$

$$= 0.545$$

$$\therefore \theta_t = \sin^{-1}(0.545)$$

$$= 33°$$

$$\text{Beam deviation} = \theta_t - \theta_i$$

$$= 3°$$

I.9 DOPPLER SHIFT (f_d), REFLECTOR VELOCITY (V), TRANSMITTED FREQUENCY (f_0), BEAM/DIRECTION OF MOVEMENT ANGLE (θ), SPEED OF ULTRASOUND (c)

Equation:

$$f_d = -\frac{2V f_0 \cos \theta}{c} \qquad (I.15)$$

Question:
Given V = −50 cm/s (towards transducers), f_0 = 5 MHz, θ = 60° and c = 1540 m/s, what is f_d?

Answer:

$$V = -50 \text{ cm/s}$$

$$= -0.5 \text{ m/s}$$

$$f_d = -\frac{2Vf_0 \cos \theta}{c}$$

$$= \frac{2 \times 0.5 \times 5 \times 10^6 \times \cos 60°}{1540} \text{ Hz}$$

$$= 1.62 \times 10^3 \text{ Hz}$$

$$= 1.62 \text{ kHz}$$

I.10 BLOOD FLOW RATE (F_1), MEAN DOPPLER SHIFT (f_d), TRANSMITTED FREQUENCY (f_0), BEAM/VESSEL ANGLE (θ), VESSEL DIAMETER (D), SPEED OF ULTRASOUND (c)

Equation:

From equation I.15:

$$V = \frac{-cf_d}{2f_0 \cos \theta} \qquad (I.16)$$

Vessel cross-sectional area $= \dfrac{\pi D^2}{4}$

$$F_1 = \text{velocity} \times \text{area}$$

$$= \frac{-cf_d \pi D^2}{8f_0 \cos \theta} \qquad (I.17)$$

Question:

Given $c = 1570$ m/s, $f_d = 1.2$ kHz, $D = 6$ mm, $f_0 = 10$ MHz and $\theta = 60°$ what is F_1?

Answer:

$$F_1 = -\frac{1570 \times 1.2 \times 10^3 \times \pi \times 0.006^2}{8 \times 10^7 \times \cos 60°}$$

$$= -5.33 \times 10^{-6} \text{ m}^3/\text{s}$$

$$= -5.33 \times 10^{-3} \text{ l/s}$$

$$= -5.33 \text{ ml/s}$$

Bibliography

Aero-Tech Reports—Ultrasonic Transducer Performance Parameters. K.B.-Aerotech, P.O. Box 350, Lewistown, PA 17044, USA.

Atkinson, P and Woodcock, J.P. (1982) Doppler Ultrasound and its Use in Clinical ·Measurement. Academic Press.

Barnett, E. and Morley, P. (1985) Clinical Diagnostic Ultrasound. Blackwell Scientific Publication.

Evans, D.H., McDicken, W.N., Skidmore, R. and Woodcock, J.P. (1989) Doppler Ultrasound. Physics, Instrumentation and Clinical Applications. Wiley.

Geigy Pharmaceutical Co. Ltd, (1962) Documents Geigy Scientific Tables. 6th Edition.

Hill, C.R. (1986) Physical Principles of Medical Ultrasonics. Ellis Horwood.

Hussey, M. (1985) Basic Physics and Technology of Medical Diagnostic Ultrasound. Macmillan.

Hykes, D., Hedrick, W.R. and Starchman, D.E. (1985) Ultrasound Physics and Instrumentation. Churchill Livingstone.

Kempczinski, R.F. and Yao, J.S.T. (1982) Practical Non-invasive Vascular Diagnosis. Year Book Medical Publishers.

Kremkau, F.W. (1989) Diagnostic Ultrasound—Principles, Instruments and Exercises, 3rd Edition W.B. Saunders.

Lerski, R.A. (1988) Practical Ultrasound. IRL Press.

McDicken, W.N. (1981) Diagnostic Ultrasonics: Principles and Use of Instruments, 2nd Edition. Wiley.

Powis, R.L. and Powis, W.J. (1984) A Thinker's Guide to Ultrasonic Imaging. Urban and Schwarzenberg.

Shirley, I.M., Blackwell, R.J., Cusick, G., Farman, D.J. and Vickary, F.R. (1978) A User's Guide to Diagnostic Ultrasound. Pitman Medical.

Taylor, K.J.W., Burns, P.N. and Wells, P.N.T. (1988) Clinical Applications of Doppler Ultrasound. Raven Press.

The College of Radiographers Certificate of Medical Ultrasound, Examiners Reports 1985–1988. The College of Radiographers, 11 Wimpole Street, London, W1M 8BN, UK.

Topping, J. (1963) Errors of Observation and their Treatment. Chapman and Hall.

Wells, P.N.T. (1977) Biomedical Ultrasonics. Academic Press.

Williams, A.R. (1983) Ultrasound: Biological Effects and Potential Hazards. Academic Press.

Woodcock, J.P. (1979) Ultrasonics. Adam Hilger.

Index